T0362298

Reproductive Health

Editors

LISA R. SAMMARITANO
ELIZA F. CHAKRAVARTY

RHEUMATIC
DISEASE CLINICS
OF NORTH AMERICA

www.rheumatic.theclinics.com

Consulting Editor
MICHAEL H. WEISMAN

May 2017 • Volume 43 • Number 2

ELSEVIER

1600 John F. Kennedy Boulevard • Suite 1800 • Philadelphia, Pennsylvania, 19103-2899
http://www.theclinics.com

RHEUMATIC DISEASE CLINICS OF NORTH AMERICA Volume 43, Number 2
May 2017 ISSN 0889-857X, ISBN 13: 978-0-323-52860-3

Editor: Lauren Boyle
Developmental Editor: Casey Potter

Rheumatic Disease Clinics of North America (ISSN 0889-857X) is published quarterly by Elsevier Inc., 360 Park Avenue South, New York, NY 10010-1710. Months of issue are February, May, August, and November. Business and editorial offices: 1600 John F. Kennedy Boulevard, Suite 1800, Philadelphia, PA 19103-2899. Periodicals postage paid at New York, NY and additional mailing offices. Subscription prices are USD 335.00 per year for US individuals, USD 659.00 per year for US institutions, USD 100.00 per year for US students and residents, USD 395.00 per year for Canadian individuals, USD 823.00 per year for Canadian institutions, USD 465.00 per year for international individuals, USD 823.00 per year for international institutions, and USD 230.00 per year for Canadian and foreign students/residents. To receive student/resident rate, orders must be accompanied by name of affiliated institution, date of term, and the *signature* of program/residency coordinator on institution letterhead. Orders will be billed at individual rate until proof of status received. Foreign air speed delivery is included in all *Clinics* subscription prices. All prices are subject to change without notice. **POSTMASTER:** Send address changes to *Rheumatic Disease Clinics of North America,* Elsevier Health Sciences Division, Subscription Customer Service, 3251 Riverport Lane, Maryland Heights, MO 63043. **Customer Service: 1-800-654-2452 (US and Canada). From outside of the US and Canada: 314-447-8871. Fax: 314-447-8029. For print support, e-mail: JournalsCustomerService-usa@elsevier.com. For online support, e-mail: JournalsOnline Support-usa@elsevier.com.**

Reprints. For copies of 100 or more of articles in this publication, please contact the Commercial Reprints Department, Elsevier Inc., 360 Park Avenue South, New York, New York, 10010-1710; Tel.: +1-212-633-3874, Fax: +1-212-633-3820, and E-mail: reprints@elsevier.com.

Rheumatic Disease Clinics of North America is covered in *MEDLINE/PubMed (Index Medicus), Current Contents/Clinical Medicine, Science Citation Index, ISI/BIOMED,* and *EMBASE/Excerpta Medica.*

Contributors

CONSULTING EDITOR

MICHAEL H. WEISMAN, MD
Cedars-Sinai Chair, Director, Division of Rheumatology, Professor of Medicine, Cedars-Sinai Medical Center, Distinguished Professor, David Geffen School of Medicine at UCLA, Los Angeles, California

EDITORS

LISA R. SAMMARITANO, MD
Associate Professor of Clinical Medicine, Hospital for Special Surgery, Weill Cornell Medicine, New York, New York

ELIZA F. CHAKRAVARTY, MD, MS
Associate Member, Division of Arthritis and Clinical Immunology, Oklahoma Medical Research Foundation, Oklahoma City, Oklahoma

AUTHORS

BONNIE L. BERMAS, MD
Clinical Director, Lupus Center, Division of Rheumatology, Immunology and Allergy, Brigham and Women's Hospital, Boston, Massachusetts

SASHA BERNATSKY, MD, PhD
Associate Professor, Divisions of Clinical Epidemiology and Rheumatology, McGill University Health Centre, Montreal, Québec, Canada

ELIZA F. CHAKRAVARTY, MD, MS
Associate Member, Division of Arthritis and Clinical Immunology, Oklahoma Medical Research Foundation, Oklahoma City, Oklahoma

MEGAN E.B. CLOWSE, MD, MPH
Associate Professor of Medicine, Division of Rheumatology, Duke University Medical Center, Durham, North Carolina

PASCAL H.P. DE JONG, MD, PhD
Department of Rheumatology, Erasmus MC, Rotterdam, The Netherlands

RADBOUD J.E.M. DOLHAIN, MD, PhD
Department of Rheumatology, Erasmus MC, Rotterdam, The Netherlands

LATISHA HEINLEN, MD, PhD
Division of Rheumatology, Oklahoma University Health Sciences Center, Oklahoma City, Oklahoma

AISHA LATEEF, MBBS, MRCP, MMed, FAMS
Division of Rheumatology, University Medicine Cluster, National University Hospital, National University Health System, Singapore

LEAH MACHEN, MD
Resident in Internal Medicine, Department of Medicine, Duke University Medical Center, Durham, North Carolina

WENDY MARDER, MD, MS
Clinical Associate Professor, Division of Rheumatology, Department of Internal Medicine; Department of Obstetrics and Gynecology, University of Michigan, Ann Arbor, Michigan

CATHERINE NELSON-PIERCY, FRCP, FRCOG
Professor of Obstetric Medicine; Queen Charlotte's & Chelsea Hospital, Imperial College Healthcare NHS Trust; Women's Health Academic Centre, King's College London, St Thomas' Hospital, London, United Kingdom

MONIKA ØSTENSEN, MD
Professor; Consultant, National Advisory Unit on Pregnancy and Rheumatic Diseases, Department of Rheumatology, National Advisory Unit on Pregnancy and Rheumatic Diseases, Trondheim University Hospital, Trondheim, Norway

MICHELLE PETRI, MD, MPH
Division of Rheumatology, Johns Hopkins Lupus Center, Johns Hopkins University School of Medicine, Baltimore, Maryland

LISA R. SAMMARITANO, MD
Associate Professor of Clinical Medicine, Hospital for Special Surgery, Weill Cornell Medicine, New York, New York

ROBERT HAL SCOFIELD, MD
Professor, Section of Endocrinology, Diabetes and Metabolism, Department of Medicine, College of Medicine, University of Oklahoma Health Sciences Center; Arthritis & Clinical Immunology Program, Oklahoma Medical Research Foundation; Medical Service, Department of Veterans Affairs Medical Center, Oklahoma City, Oklahoma

MAY CHING SOH, FRACP
Consultant Physician in Obstetric Medicine; John Radcliffe Hospital, Oxford University Hospitals NHS Foundation Trust, Oxford; Queen Charlotte's & Chelsea Hospital, Imperial College Healthcare NHS Trust, Du Cane Road, London; Women's Health Academic Centre, King's College London, St Thomas' Hospital, London, United Kingdom

EMILY C. SOMERS, PhD, ScM
Associate Professor, Division of Rheumatology, Department of Internal Medicine; Department of Obstetrics and Gynecology; Department of Environmental Health Sciences, University of Michigan, Ann Arbor, Michigan

MITALI TALSANIA, MBBS
Assistant Professor, Section of Endocrinology, Diabetes and Metabolism, Department of Medicine, College of Medicine, University of Oklahoma Health Sciences Center, Oklahoma City, Oklahoma

ÉVELYNE VINET, MD, PhD
Assistant Professor, Divisions of Clinical Epidemiology and Rheumatology, McGill University Health Centre, Montreal, Québec, Canada

Contents

Although the female predominance of autoimmune diseases is not completely understood, sex hormones are thought to play a role. Attention to lifelong reproductive health is especially important for women with autoimmune disorders. Many of these women require long-term immunosuppressive therapy that may affect their ability to clear infections, including viruses, and may alter natural tumor surveillance mechanisms. As a result, women with autoimmune diseases may have different risks for common reproductive-related malignancies that may in turn affect screening guidelines and other preventive measures, including vaccination. Women with autoimmune diseases need to adhere diligently to screening recommendations.

Contraception represents an important area of reproductive health for patients with rheumatic diseases given the potential pregnancy risks associated with active disease, teratogenic medications, and severe disease-related damage. A high proportion of patients with rheumatic disease do not use effective contraception. Long-acting contraceptives are most effective. Antiphospholipid-negative patients with stable systemic lupus erythematosus may use oral combined contraceptives. Antiphospholipid-positive patients, or patients with rheumatic disease with other risk factors for thrombosis, should avoid estrogen-containing contraceptives. Contraceptive methods should be addressed by both the rheumatologist and gynecologist to determine the safest, most effective, and most convenient form for each patient.

Chronic rheumatic disease may interfere with procreation in women of childbearing age. Female patients should have counseling in regard to family planning and parenting. Preconception counseling requires risk assessment of possible maternal or fetal risks, screening for biomarkers with predictive value for adverse pregnancy outcomes, adjustment of therapy, and a schedule for monitoring and follow-up during pregnancy. Delivering comprehensive information and addressing all patient concerns are both essential for enabling patients to engage actively in decision making.

May Ching Soh and Catherine Nelson-Piercy

Pregnancy is a delicate balance of angiogenic factors. Adverse pregnancy outcomes in the form of placental insufficiency occur when antiangiogenic factors predominate, which manifests as maternal-placental syndrome (MPS). Women with rheumatic disease are at increased risk of MPS. Endothelial damage from circulating antiangiogenic factors and other inflammatory molecules in combination with preexisting maternal vascular risk factors is the likely underlying pathophysiological process for MPS. It is likely that these changes persist, and additional "insults" from ongoing inflammation, medications, and disease damage contribute to the development of accelerated cardiovascular disease seen in young women with rheumatic disease.

Aisha Lateef and Michelle Petri

Systemic lupus erythematosus (SLE) is an autoimmune disease with a strong female predilection. Pregnancy remains a commonly encountered but high-risk situation in this setting. Both maternal and fetal mortality and morbidity are still significantly increased despite improvements in outcomes. Maternal morbidity includes higher risk of disease flares, preeclampsia and other pregnancy-related complications. Fetal issues include higher rates of preterm birth, intrauterine growth restriction, and neonatal lupus syndromes. Treatment options during pregnancy are also limited and maternal benefit has to be weighed against fetal risk. A coordinated approach, with close monitoring by a multidisciplinary team, is essential for optimal outcomes.

Pascal H.P. de Jong and Radboud J.E.M. Dolhain

Fertility is impaired in women with rheumatoid arthritis (RA), whereas less is known about male fertility problems. Pregnancy outcome in patients with RA is slightly less favorable compared with the general population, especially in patients with active disease. Disease activity usually improves during pregnancy, but less than previously thought. Although several antirheumatic drugs are contraindicated in pregnancy, more treatment options are available. There is evidence on the safety of TNF inhibitors in pregnancy. Given the impact of active disease on fertility and pregnancy outcome, a treat-to-target strategy is recommended for patients who are pregnant or have a wish to conceive.

Leah Machen and Megan E.B. Clowse

Vasculitis is more often a disease of women beyond their reproductive years, leaving the challenges of pregnancy management difficult to study.

Pregnancy complications, including pregnancy loss and preterm birth, are higher among women with all forms of vasculitis. It seems that controlling the disease before pregnancy may improve the chances of pregnancy success. Many medications used for vasculitis are considered low risk in pregnancy, including prednisone, colchicine, azathioprine, and tumor necrosis factor inhibitors. Cyclophosphamide, methotrexate, and mycophenolate mofetil should be avoided in pregnancy. Controlling disease with low-risk medications may allow women with vasculitis to have the pregnancies they desire.

While much of the existing literature in the field of reproductive rheumatology focuses on fertility, preconception counseling, and pregnancy, there is limited information regarding the postpartum period and lactation. Evidence suggests that many rheumatologic disorders flare after delivery, which, along with limitations in medications compatible with breastfeeding, make this time period challenging for women with rheumatologic conditions. This article discusses rheumatologic disease activity during the postpartum period and reviews the safety during lactation of commonly used medications for the management of rheumatic diseases. Fortunately, many of the commonly used medications are compatible with breastfeeding.

Systemic lupus erythematosus (SLE) and rheumatoid arthritis (RA) are the most prevalent autoimmune rheumatic diseases, predominantly occurring in women during childbearing years. Research has focused on assessing the risk of immediate complications during SLE and RA pregnancies, with studies documenting a higher risk of adverse obstetric outcomes, such as preterm births and infants small for gestational age. Until recently, little was known regarding the long-term health of children born to affected women. We present a review of the current evidence regarding the risk of adverse health outcomes in SLE and RA offspring, and potential mechanisms involved in their pathogenesis.

Infertility and subfertility, menstrual irregularities, and decreased parity may occur in women with autoimmune diseases due to multiple factors, including underlying inflammatory disease, gonadotoxic medications, and psychosocial issues related to living with chronic disease. Awareness of these factors, as well as validation and support of patients confronting reproductive challenges, is important for providing comprehensive care to these women. An understanding of the expanding options for fertility preservation strategies during gonadotoxic medications is essential. Referral to a reproductive endocrinology clinic is indicated in this patient population.

Mitali Talsania and Robert Hal Scofield

Menopause occurs naturally in women at about 50 years of age. There is a wealth of data concerning the relationship of menopause to systemic lupus erythematosus, rheumatoid arthritis, and osteoarthritis; there are limited data concerning other rheumatic diseases. Age at menopause may affect the risk and course of rheumatic diseases. Osteoporosis, an integral part of inflammatory rheumatic diseases, is made worse by menopause. Hormone replacement therapy has been studied; its effects vary depending on the disease and even different manifestations within the same disease. Cyclophosphamide can induce early menopause, but there is underlying decreased ovarian reserve in rheumatic diseases.

RHEUMATIC DISEASE CLINICS
OF NORTH AMERICA

THE CLINICS ARE AVAILABLE ONLINE!
Access your subscription at:
www.theclinics.com

Foreword

Reproductive Health

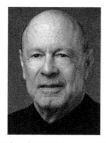

Michael H. Weisman, MD
Consulting Editor

Lisa Sammaritano and Eliza Chakravarty have put together a remarkable issue summarizing state-of-the-art knowledge of diagnosis, pathogenesis, management, and prevention in the important world of reproductive health. Both editors have assembled an impressive array of talent to take us through an in-depth approach. Lisa herself has addressed the complex area of contraception in our patients with rheumatic diseases, emphasizing the need for a proper balance between the high risk (to both mother and child) of pregnancy and the risk of methods to prevent it. Bonnie Bermas follows this article, addressing the common theme of medication implementation to avoid disease flare and possible risk to the newborn contrasted with the clear benefits of breastfeeding for both mother and child. Monica Ostensen discusses the overall important concept of medication risk worries and the benefits of optimal disease control. She addresses the ideal situation where preconception counseling should be shared with all doctors and health professionals involved in the care of a pregnant patient. De Jong and Dolhain get right to the point through their emphasis on optimal control of disease activity in order to counter the data that rheumatoid arthritis pregnancy outcomes are less favorable compared with the general population; they postulate that this is most likely related to incomplete control of disease activity. These authors discuss emerging evidence on the safety of TNF inhibitors in the pregnant RA patient. Megan Clowse, a senior authority in this complex area, discusses the interplay between vasculitis disease activity management with potentially teratogenic medications and pregnancy outcome. She emphasizes that commonly employed medications used to treat various forms of vasculitis (methotrexate, cyclophosphamide, and mycophenolate) are teratogenic and should be replaced in the pregnant patient with lower-risk alternatives.

Vinet and Bernatsky provide a thoughtful epidemiologic approach to the widely disparate data on pregnancy outcomes and address the small but significant risk to optimal pregnancy outcomes in our RA and SLE patients. They point out that the absolute risk is small and by itself should not be an automatic discouragement to having children. Somers and Marder tackle the ever-present problem of fertility in the face of

Rheum Dis Clin N Am 43 (2017) xi–xii
http://dx.doi.org/10.1016/j.rdc.2017.02.002
0889-857X/17/© 2017 Published by Elsevier Inc.

rheumatic.theclinics.com

the disease itself as well as medications used to control the disease and their effect on preservation of ovarian function. Significant advances have been made in this area. Soh and Nelson-Piercy discuss the emerging role of biomarkers to assign risk for pre-eclampsia or accelerated cardiovascular risk in young women with rheumatic diseases; they caution about overinterpretation of rapidly accumulating data and oversimplification of a complex clinical problem. Lateef and Petri, with a wealth of SLE experience, recommend specific monitoring protocols and very closely tailored multidisciplinary care to avoid unwanted outcomes to mother and child. Heinlin and Chakravarty thoughtfully review the risks and development of comorbid conditions, including cancer in women with systemic autoimmune diseases, and Talsania and Scofield discuss the complex interplay between physiologic menopause and both susceptibility and severity of several rheumatic diseases.

It is hoped this issue will stimulate others to move the field forward by pointing out the advantages of a comprehensive approach to the clinical care of these patients as well as the need to stimulate investigators to provide much needed insights where there are gaps in our knowledge. These editors deserve congratulations on a job well done.

Michael H. Weisman, MD
Division of Rheumatology
Cedars-Sinai Medical Center
David Geffen School of Medicine at UCLA
8700 Beverly Boulevard
Los Angeles, CA 90024, USA

E-mail address:
Michael.Weisman@cshs.org

Preface

Reproductive Rheumatology: Meeting Today's Challenges

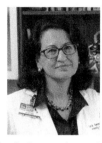 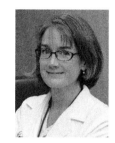

Lisa R. Sammaritano, MD   Eliza F. Chakravarty, MD, MS
Editors

It has been a delight to organize and edit this compilation of articles summarizing the current knowledge and future directions of reproductive health in women with systemic rheumatic diseases. We are indebted to all of the authors worldwide who have contributed such outstanding articles to this issue of *Rheumatic Disease Clinics of North America*.

Women make up the majority of patients with systemic rheumatic diseases. With advances in the diagnosis and treatment of underlying rheumatic disease, patients have both improved life expectancy and quality of life: many now feel healthy enough to consider and desire pregnancy and childrearing. Rheumatologists caring for these women must now consider contraception, pregnancy, lactation, reproductive health care screening, and menopause when providing longitudinal care. The interrelationships between female sex hormones and underlying rheumatic disease are complex and remain incompletely understood. However, the last few decades have provided a foundation of clinical data to guide the clinician regarding medical management of rheumatic disease through the female reproductive lifespan with particular emphasis on balancing risks of untreated or undertreated disease on pregnancy outcomes with the potential risks of immunosuppressive therapy as well as hormonal therapy. Reproductive health care for women with rheumatic diseases goes well beyond risk stratification and medical management throughout pregnancy and includes issues such as safe and effective contraception, infertility and fertility therapies, human papilloma virus, menopause, and developing fields of study, such as monitoring offspring of women with rheumatic diseases beyond the immediate neonatal period into childhood and beyond.

We have been fortunate to assemble a group of contributors whose work over the past few decades has significantly contributed to the growing field of reproductive rheumatology and makes up the basis for many of the recommendations discussed in this issue. Much of the data, particularly on use of medications to treat rheumatic

Rheum Dis Clin N Am 43 (2017) xiii–xiv
http://dx.doi.org/10.1016/j.rdc.2017.02.001
0889-857X/17/© 2017 Published by Elsevier Inc.

rheumatic.theclinics.com

diseases during pregnancy, remains somewhat controversial; therefore, some recommendations will vary slightly between different authors. This is a reflection of differing expert opinions based on the relatively limited clinical data that are currently available. We anticipate and hope that, given the complex immunology involved as well as the need for more definitive clinical data, research on reproductive issues within rheumatology will continue to expand and attract young investigators.

We would like to thank all of the authors for their outstanding contributions and hope that readers will find this information valuable in guiding truly comprehensive care for women with rheumatic diseases.

Lisa R. Sammaritano, MD
Weill Cornell Medicine
Hospital for Special Surgery
535 East 70th Street
New York, NY 10021, USA

Eliza F. Chakravarty, MD, MS
Arthritis and Clinical Immunology
Oklahoma Medical Research Foundation
825 NE 13th Street
Oklahoma City, OK 73104, USA

E-mail addresses:
sammaritanol@hss.edu (L.R. Sammaritano)
chakravartye@omrf.org (E.F. Chakravarty)

Reproductive Health Screening in Women with Autoimmune Diseases

Latisha Heinlen, MD, PhD[a], Eliza F. Chakravarty, MD, MS[b],*

KEYWORDS

- Autoimmune diseases • Rheumatoid arthritis • Systemic lupus erythematosus
- Breast cancer • Cervical cancer • Human papilloma virus • Preventive health
- Screening

KEY POINTS

- Advances in treatment of autoimmune diseases have led to a reduction in mortality and increased quality of life for these patients, making issues related to long-term preventive health and aging more relevant.
- Immune dysregulation from immunosuppressant medications or the underlying diseases may affect clearance of viral infections or innate tumor surveillance among people with autoimmune diseases.
- Breast cancer risk does not seem to be increased among women with rheumatoid arthritis or systemic lupus erythematosus compared with the general female population.
- Studies are conflicting regarding the relative risk of invasive cervical cancer in women with autoimmune diseases, but there is concern for increased rates of precancerous lesions, including cervical dysplasia and atypia, for which early treatment may affect the development of invasive cancer.

INTRODUCTION

It is well known that many systemic autoimmune diseases, including systemic lupus erythematosus (SLE) and rheumatoid arthritis (RA), carry a striking female predominance. Reasons for this are thought to be multifactorial, but likely involve interrelationships between female sex hormones and the immune system. Because of this correlation, there is concern about the influence of autoimmune disease on the reproductive health of affected women. Aside from well-studied influences of underlying disease on pregnancy, there remains concern that common triggering factors may

[a] Division of Rheumatology, Oklahoma University Health Sciences Center, 1100 N. Lindsay Avenue, Oklahoma City, OK 73104, USA; [b] Division of Arthritis and Clinical Immunology; Oklahoma Medical Research Foundation, 825 Northeast 13th Street, Oklahoma City, OK 73104, USA
* Corresponding author.
E-mail address: chakravartye@omrf.org

Rheum Dis Clin N Am 43 (2017) 161–171
http://dx.doi.org/10.1016/j.rdc.2016.12.010
0889-857X/17/© 2017 Elsevier Inc. All rights reserved.

influence the development of both autoimmune disease and hormonal malignancies. There is additional concern that the presence of autoimmunity or chronic immunosuppressive medication may mediate risk of chronic viral infections, including human papilloma virus (HPV), known to cause cervical and other malignancies.

Required reporting of invasive cancers to national cancer registries has allowed the estimation of site-specific malignancies by age, race, and gender in the general population. By studying rates observed in large cohorts of autoimmune diseases, standardized incidence ratios (SIRs; the ratio of observed cancers to those expected based on age and gender norms) can be calculated to study the rates of cancer, including female malignancies, providing an easy reference of relative risk of these malignancies that may influence screening practices. This method has been widely used to study the changes in risk of hematologic malignancies and lymphoma in patients with RA who use tumor necrosis factor (TNF) inhibitor medications.

Given increased survival rates and improved disease management for many patients with RA and SLE, attention to the risks and development of comorbid conditions, including cancer, has become more important for patients and their providers. Relative risks of hormone-based malignancies, as well as the identification of specific disease-related or medication-related risks, are critical when caring for women with autoimmune disease across their lifespan so that appropriate screening and preventive services can be implemented as part of comprehensive health care. Admittedly, many patients with underlying systemic autoimmune diseases see their rheumatologists for management of active disease manifestations, and minimization of medication toxicities and/or visits to primary care or other preventive health services may become less prioritized. It is important to understand the rates of breast and cervical cancers in women with SLE and RA, risk factors for development of malignancies, and appropriate screening procedures. The addition of a primary care provider to the medical team may greatly enhance adherence to preventive screening for cancer as well as other comorbid conditions that could complicate underlying autoimmune disease.

BREAST CANCER

Breast cancer is the most common malignancy seen in the general female population, with approximately 1.7 million cases diagnosed worldwide in 2012. Known risk factors for the development of breast cancer include family history, age, race, parity, breastfeeding, use of exogenous estrogens, alcohol, sedentary lifestyle, and increased body mass index.[1] Given that autoimmune diseases often preferentially affect women and may bear unique relationships with female sex hormones, it is important to understand the relative risk of breast cancer among women affected by these chronic diseases. Several large multinational studies have been performed to compare rates of numerous types of cancers in patients with autoimmune diseases and the general population. For example, it is well known that many autoimmune diseases increase the risk of lymphoma compared with the general population, although the absolute risk remains low.

Breast Cancer and Systemic Lupus Erythematosus

Several large studies and meta-analyses have been published to examine the SIR of breast cancer in women with SLE. One of the largest studies was performed by the international Systemic Lupus International Collaborating Clinics (SLICC), in which 16,000 patients with SLE from 30 participating centers were followed longitudinally. A total of 180 cases of breast cancer were reported: the average age at diagnosis was 54 years, which is younger than the mean of 60 years in the general population, with a mean SLE duration of 14 years.[2] The SIR of overall breast cancer in this SLE population was 0.73 (95% confidence interval [CI], 0.61–0.88), indicating a lower than expected incidence of breast cancer in SLE.[3] A separate group performed an analysis of breast cancer incidence among women with or without SLE enrolled in a population-based study of US Medicare recipients.[4] A cohort of 18,423 women with a diagnosis of SLE was compared with 3,651,715 women without SLE. The 5-year age-adjusted incidence risk for patients with SLE overall was 2.23 (95% CI, 1.94–2.55) per 100 women compared with 2.59 (95% CI, 2.57–2.61) among women without SLE, with an overall unadjusted risk ratio of 0.87 (95% CI, 0.79–0.86), confirming the SLICC results showing no increased risk of breast cancer. These results were similar when examining breast cancer risk in subgroups of women by race or age (older or younger than 65 years). Furthermore, a separate study of the United States Renal Data System evaluated site-specific cancer risk in renal transplant recipients, comparing rates of cancer in 4289 transplant recipients with SLE versus 139,363 transplant recipients without SLE with what would be expected in the general population.[5] The overall SIR for cancer was increased for all transplant recipients by approximately 3-fold: 3.5 (95% CI, 2.1–5.7) for SLE and 3.7 (95% CI, 2.4–5.7) for non-SLE. Similarly, breast cancer showed an increased incidence in all transplant recipients by approximately 2-fold, but this was not different between patients with and without SLE, suggesting that the increased risk of breast cancer may be related more to end-stage renal disease, dialysis, and transplantation rather than SLE-specific factors.

In order to better understand demographic and disease-related risk factors for breast cancer among women with SLE, the SLICC group performed a case-cohort analyses of a subset of the patients with SLE who developed breast cancer compared with cancer-free patients with SLE.[6] Eighty-six women with SLE diagnosed with breast cancer were compared with 4498 cancer-free women with SLE. Women with breast cancer were older than the cancer-free controls and more likely to be white (81% vs 62%). There were no significant differences in disease activity over time or autoantibody prevalence between the groups. In univariate analyses, only age, white ancestry, menopausal status, postmenopausal hormone therapy, and family history of breast cancer were associated with breast cancer risk, which is similar to what is seen in the general population. However, in multivariable analysis, only increasing age remained statistically significant. Variables related to SLE disease activity, autoantibody prevalence, or medication use were not associated with breast cancer risk in this international cohort.[6] Thus, although some data suggest a possible decreased risk of breast cancer among patients with SLE, other data suggest it is similar. To date, no disease-related factors seem to mitigate breast cancer risk in women with SLE. Male breast cancer in SLE has not been systematically studied.

Rheumatoid Arthritis and Breast Cancer

Similar to SLE, overall malignancy rates for RA seem to be slightly increased compared with the general population, with most of the increases seen in the hematologic malignancies. Also like SLE, rates of breast cancer among women with RA seem to be lower than what is expected based on age and ethnicity. The introduction and widespread use of biologic therapies for RA have changed clinical practice since the turn of the century. Given the addition of biologic therapies and the possibility of affecting rates of malignancies seen in patients with RA, a recent meta-analysis was performed evaluating studies published from 2008 to 2014.[7] The pooled SIR for breast cancer in this meta-analysis of 0.84 (95% CI, 0.73–1.01) was similar to the pooled SIR found in an earlier meta-analysis (pre–biologic therapy use) of 0.83

(95% CI, 0.79–0.90),[8] the main change being that the CI now crosses the null. Therefore, the conclusion that breast cancer risk does not seem to be increased in women with RA is upheld even with the addition of different RA treatment strategies, although the decrease in rate is no longer consistent. A separate meta-analysis, isolated to breast cancer in RA, was performed that showed consistent results of a numerically decreased rate of breast cancer compared with the general population.[9] However, this study went further to evaluate breast cancer risk by ethnicity, identifying an increased risk for breast cancer among nonwhite women with RA compared with the general population. The slightly reduced risk of breast cancer among white women with RA was similar to that seen in the overall RA population.

Given the concern about reduced tumor surveillance with the use of TNF antagonists, there has been hesitancy for initiating these agents in patients with RA with a remote history of breast cancer. Two studies have been recently been published to evaluate the change in risk to women with RA with a history of breast cancer who begin therapy with TNF antagonists.[10,11] The first study evaluated a cohort of 143 Swedish patients with RA with a history of breast cancer who were later initiated on TNF antagonist therapy and compared them with 143 (out of a total of 1598) patients with RA with a history of breast cancer who were not treated with biologic therapy.[10] Subjects were matched on sex, age at cancer diagnosis, year of cancer diagnosis, and stage of cancer at diagnosis, and were followed for approximately 5 years for breast cancer recurrence. Patients who started TNF therapy did so after approximately 9 years from original cancer diagnosis, generally following previous guidelines to wait at least 5 years before initiating biologic therapy. The study did not find an increased risk of breast cancer recurrence between groups, with a hazard ratio of 0.8 (95% CI, 0.3–2.1), although the sample size was small. These data were supported by a larger study of breast cancer recurrence in a Medicare population including women with RA or inflammatory bowel disease.[11] The larger population (a total of 2684 women) under study allowed for an analysis not only of the effects of TNF inhibition on cancer recurrence but also of other commonly used immunosuppressive medications, including methotrexate and thiopurines. Women with each exposure were matched to a cohort of women without the medication exposure and were analyzed separately. Numerically, the hazard ratio was increased for users of all 3 therapies compared with nonusers, but the CIs were wide and crossed the null, therefore not establishing a statistically significant increase. Many of these women initiated immunosuppressive therapy for autoimmune disease before or shortly following initial diagnosis of breast cancer. Thus, a history of breast cancer should not necessarily preclude the use of traditional disease-modifying antirheumatic drugs (DMARDs) or biologic therapies for management of active RA.

Recommendations for Screening for Breast Cancer

Despite some data suggesting a possible decreased incidence of breast cancer in women with RA compared with the general population, women with RA should not think themselves protected from developing one of the most common cancers among women worldwide, nor should they develop a sense of complacency regarding routine health screening for breast cancer. The main risk factors for breast cancer for women with RA are not different from those of women without RA: increasing age, family history, menopausal status, and use of postmenopausal hormone therapy are among the most important risk factors. Women with RA should follow the same screening recommendations as women without RA regarding breast cancer, based on the presence and number of risk factors. Similar to the general population, any palpable, visual, or radiographic changes to the breast that raise suspicion for breast cancer should prompt a thorough evaluation.

CERVICAL CANCER

Cervical cancer, a virus-associated malignancy, has been studied in autoimmune disease to determine whether the risk is increased owing to immune suppression as well as underlying immune dysfunction. Patients with RA analyzed in a Canadian population did not have an increase in cervical cancer when analyzed retrospectively,[12] although later studies of patients with RA in California did show an increased risk of malignancy, including cervical cancer.[13] Chang and colleagues[14] found no increase in incidence of cervical cancer in patients with RA, scleroderma, or myositis, whereas they did find an increased risk in patients with SLE. Although the risk of malignancy is thought to be increased in autoimmune disease, as suggested by these studies, there may be significant geographic differences in risk for specific malignancies.

Cervical cancer as well as cervical dysplasia has long been shown to be increased in patients with SLE. This increase was initially recognized in a Swedish study in 1981, in which Nyberg and colleagues[15] found an increased risk in patients with SLE who had received chemotherapy. Subsequent studies have consistently shown an increased risk for cervical atypia in patients with SLE that seems to be increased further with immune suppression.[16–18] Cibere and colleagues[19] followed 297 Canadian patients with SLE for up to 10 years and found that cervical cancer was significantly increased compared with controls (SIR = 8.15; 95% CI, 1.63–23.81), although the number of cases was low with only 3 diagnosed cases. Recently, large retrospective studies using the Korean National Cancer Registry have shown an increase in cervical cancer in patients with SLE compared with controls (SIR = 4.28; 95% CI, 1.72–8.82).[14] Increased risk of cervical cancer in patients with SLE varies by the population studied; in a recent meta-analysis, the increased risk was evaluated using 7 previously published studies and a total of 445 cases and 3379 controls. The common odds ratio calculated was 4.17 (95% CI, 3.03–5.74; $P<.00001$).[20]

Cervical Cancer and Immunosuppressive Agents

Recently, because more extensive immune suppression and the addition of biologic agents have become increasingly common, this issue has been revisited because of the concern about increased malignancy caused by further immune suppression. Waisberg and colleagues[21] initially analyzed 50 patients with RA using anti-TNF therapy to determine whether there was an increased risk of HPV and *Chlamydia trachomatis* (CT) infections in this population. Patients and matched controls were screened for HPV and CT by DNA testing of cervical specimens before anti-TNF therapy as well as 6 months after treatment initiation. The investigators found no evidence of increased risk of new infection with HPV or CT, although the study was completed over a short time period. A nationwide cohort study in Sweden found that patients with RA were at higher risk of developing cervical dysplasia regardless of treatment used for their RA; however, cervical intraepithelial neoplasia grade 2-3 and invasive cervical cancer were increased in patients who used anti-TNF therapy compared with biologic-naive patients with RA.[22] Note that, when the analysis was limited to a more recent time frame (2006–2012), this association was not confirmed, perhaps because of changes in screening trends or interventions such as vaccination. A larger cohort of Danish patients showed no increased risk of cervical cancer in patients who had ever been treated with a DMARD compared with patients never treated with DMARDs.[23] In addition, Kim and colleagues[24] studied this question in a United States population and also found no difference in high-grade cervical dysplasia or cervical cancer in patients with RA started on biologic DMARD therapy. Although there are no large studies analyzing current immunosuppression regimens, previous Cytoxan use has been found to increase the risk of cervical cancer in patients with SLE and decrease the time to dysplasia in patients with HPV, although this was not confirmed in a smaller, more recent cohort.[25,26]

Systemic Lupus Erythematosus and Human Papilloma Virus Infection

The prevalence of HPV, the causal agent of cervical cancer, has been extensively studied in patients with SLE. One of the first large studies of HPV infection in patients with SLE was performed on a Chinese population and followed 144 patients prospectively.[27] The investigators found an increase in HPV infection in patients with SLE (25% were infected after 3 years; $P = .006$). Klumb and colleagues[28] isolated cervical samples from patients with SLE and controls in Brazil and analyzed for HPV DNA by polymerase chain reaction, which included HPV genotyping. Patients with SLE had a 3-fold increase in HPV infections, although they had a lower number of the classic risk factors compared with controls. There was no statistical difference between patients with lupus taking immunosuppressive medications and those who were not. However, this was not the primary aim of the study, so it may not have been powered appropriately; alternatively, the increase in HPV could be a result of intrinsic immune dysregulation caused by SLE.

Vaccination Against Human Papilloma Virus

Since 2006 a vaccine has been commercially available for vaccination of women against HPV high-risk subtypes. There are now 2 vaccines available, a quadrivalent vaccine (Gardasil, Merck) and the bivalent vaccine (Cervarix, GlaxoSmithKline). These vaccines both include HPV subtypes 16 and 18, which are responsible for 70% of cervical cancer. A new 9-valent vaccine includes 5 additional oncogenic types (31, 33, 45, 52, and 58) and should increase the protection against cervical cancer to 90%[29]; this was US Food and Drug Administration approved in 2014 for girls and women aged 9 to 26 years and boys and men aged 9 to 15 years. In addition, the Advisory Committee on Immunization Practices recently recommended addition of the 9-valent vaccine to the vaccines acceptable for routine prevention of HPV.[30] Given the increased risk of HPV infection in patients with autoimmune disease, most extensively studied in SLE, the safety and efficacy of HPV vaccination is an important consideration in these patients.

The European Union League Against Rheumatism (EULAR) has published general recommendations for vaccination in patients with autoimmune rheumatic disease and states that nonlive vaccines can be administered independent of medication use. These recommendations focus on the safety of vaccination. However, because effective vaccination depends on a robust immune system to provide adequate antibody and memory responses, researchers have questioned whether patients with autoimmune disease are able to make such responses. Immune suppression medications have not shown a decrease in responsiveness to vaccines, with the exception of rituximab, which does dramatically impair the response to vaccination.[31]

Specifically, EULAR recommends vaccination of patients with rheumatic disease for HPV, although it notes that there may be an increased risk of deep venous thrombosis (DVT). The guidelines specifically note that patients with DVT were analyzed and 90% had at least 1 traditional risk factor for DVT. In addition, current evidence of more than 900,000 girls with HPV vaccination has not shown any association with DVT. Two studies have analyzed the safety and efficacy of the HPV vaccine in patients with SLE with the quadrivalent vaccine.[32,33] The largest of these studies included 50 patients with SLE and 50 controls. After 12 months the seroconversion rates in both groups were more than 90% for antibodies against HPV 16 and 18. Furthermore, the investigators found no evidence of increased disease flare or adverse side effects in patients with SLE after receiving the vaccine.[32]

Following the widespread administration of HPV vaccines, there have been case reports of SLE developing after immunization with HPV and a causal link has been questioned. The initial case reports were of 3 patients, 1 of whom was a 17-year-old girl diagnosed with SLE 2 months after she completed HPV vaccination, and the other 2 patents had previously diagnosed autoimmune conditions but after receiving vaccination had significant flares of SLE.[34] It is also important to note that the 2 patients with disease flares after vaccination were aged 45 and 58 years, ages that are well outside the recommended HPV vaccination age range. An additional case report was recently published showing that a 15-year-old girl was diagnosed with SLE shortly after her second dose of HPV vaccine.[35] These 4 case reports describe a temporal association of vaccination followed by SLE diagnosis or flare. In contrast, a large population-based study of HPV vaccination in more than 900,000 girls found no increased risk of developing SLE after vaccination.[36]

Screening Recommendations for Autoimmune Patients

Because patients with autoimmune disease, and specifically SLE, have a higher risk of HPV infection, cervical cancer screening guidelines should be closely followed in these patients. The United States Preventive Services Task Force recommends women aged 21 to 65 years have screening Pap smear every 3 years or, for women aged 30 to 65 years, Pap smear may be combined with HPV testing, which extends the screening interval to every 5 years. Kim and colleagues[37] analyzed patients from large US commercial insurance companies and found that, in this cohort, patients with a diagnosis of RA were more likely to have appropriate cervical cancer, breast cancer, and colon cancer screening. Note that although the screening was increased in this group of high-risk individuals, it was still estimated that only 70% to 80% met the recommended cervical cancer screening goal of every 3 years. Furthermore, this study only included patients with commercial insurance and did not include patients with Medicaid or no insurance, who are much less likely to have appropriate screening.

ADHERENCE AND BARRIERS TO REPRODUCTIVE HEALTH SCREENING

Patients with chronic autoimmune diseases have high health care use rates because of acute management of changing disease activity and monitoring for medication toxicity. In addition, providers and patients alike are becoming increasingly aware of increased risks of cardiovascular disease, stroke, osteoporosis, and infection compared with age-matched healthy individuals. Health care maintenance and screening for other conditions, however prevalent in the general population, may become a lower priority. However, the question that remains, is how to ensure that screening guidelines for female reproductive health are being met. When a woman is of child-bearing potential, reproductive health screening can occur at the same time as contraception counseling. However, studies have shown that even women of childbearing potential who are receiving teratogenic medications have surprisingly low rates of documented contraceptive counseling and use of effective contraceptive methods.[38] These low rates are especially concerning given the immediacy and potential severity of an unintended pregnancy, and rates of adherence to screening guidelines are likely to be significantly lower for conditions with a lower and more remote potential of occurrence, and for which the screening procedures are uncomfortable (pelvic examinations and mammography). Published studies of adherence to reproductive malignancy screening guidelines for women with autoimmune diseases remain scarce. For RA, several earlier studies suggested that individuals with the disease had lower rates of reproductive health screening than did the general population,[39–41] although a more recent study of individuals covered by a large US commercial insurance plan showed rates similar or even better among patients with RA compared with patients without RA,[37] suggesting that access to care and insurance coverage are critical components to comprehensive health care.

Similarly, studies of patients with SLE have shown that socioeconomic status and health care coverage play significant roles in reproductive screening rates. A study of 685 female SLE participants in the Lupus Outcomes Study in California found similar rates of cervical cancer screening and mammography (approximately 70%) among patients with SLE compared with the general population in California. Most of this cohort were well educated (completed high school), insured, and not living in high-poverty neighborhoods.[42] A cross-sectional study of a population-based cohort of patients with SLE in Atlanta, Georgia, found high rates of cervical cancer screening and mammography (>80%) among patients with SLE, similar to rates in the community.[43] Like the California study, lower screening rates were associated with younger age, poverty, and health insurance status. However, many patients with RA or SLE have lower socioeconomic status, are often not working, and have more limited access to health care and comprehensive health care coverage, placing them at higher risk for missing suggested screening practices. Adherence to cancer screening was higher in these populations than adherence to other preventive health services, including immunizations and cardiovascular risk factor monitoring. Taken together, these studies suggest not only that access to health care is critical for adherence to screening guidelines but also specifically that patients need access to a primary care provider who will focus on elements of health outside of those that are directly related to management of rheumatic disease activity.[42]

SUMMARY

Women with systemic autoimmune diseases face many challenges, and management of active disease and medication toxicity often takes primacy in health care interactions for such conditions. However, because disease-modifying agents have afforded many patients a reduction in disability and improved lifespan, issues of preventive health care and reducing the burden of comorbidities become ever more relevant. Guidelines exist for screening for reproductive malignancies that are common in the population and for which screening has been shown to decrease mortality from the diseases, including breast and cervical cancer. Several large, well-done cohort studies have shown that rates of breast and cervical cancer do not seem to be increased in women with RA or SLE compared with those that would be expected in the general population, and that risk assessment for these malignancies should be based on the presence of traditional risk factors, including age and family history. However, it is important to recognize that although rates of these malignancies do not seem to be higher than in the general population, there does not seem to be a significant protective factor afforded by autoimmune disease that reduces the rates considerably. Therefore, the best way to minimize morbidity and mortality from breast and cervical cancers is to adhere to published screening and HPV vaccination guidelines. Age, socioeconomic, and insurance factors, among other preventive health services, all seem to reduce rates of cancer screening. In contrast, having a primary care provider or generalist as part of the health care team, whose role is to manage preventive health care, seems to improve adherence to guidelines and should be implemented whenever possible.

REFERENCES

1. Rudolph A, Chang-Claude J, Schmidt MK. Gene-environment interaction and risk of breast cancer. Br J Cancer 2016;114:125–33.
2. Cloutier BT, Clarke AE, Ramsey-Goldman R, et al. Breast cancer in systemic lupus erythematosus. Oncology 2013;85:117–21.
3. Bernatsky S, Ramsey-Goldman R, Labrecque J, et al. Cancer risk in systemic lupus: an updated international multi-center cohort study. J Autoimmun 2013; 42:130–5.
4. Khaliq W, Qayyum R, Clough J, et al. Comparison of breast cancer risk in women with and without systemic lupus erythematosus in a Medicare population. Breast Cancer Res Treat 2015;151:465–74.
5. Ramsey-Goldman R, Brar A, Richardson C, et al. Standardised incidence ratios (SIRs) for cancer after renal transplantation in systemic lupus erythematosus (SLE) and non-SLE recipients. Lupus Sci Med 2016;3(1):e000156.
6. Bernatsky S, Ramsay-Goldman R, Petri M, et al. Breast cancer in systemic lupus. Lupus 2017;26(3):311–5.
7. Simon TA, Thompson A, Gandhi KK, et al. Incidence of malignancy in adult patients with rheumatoid arthritis: a meta-analysis. Arthritis Res Ther 2015;17:212.
8. Smitten AL, Simon TA, Hochberg MC, et al. A meta-analysis of the incidence of malignancy in adult patients with rheumatoid arthritis. Arthritis Res Ther 2008; 10:R45.
9. Tian G, Liang JN, Wang ZY, et al. Breast cancer risk in rheumatoid arthritis: an update meta-analysis. Biomed Res Int 2014;2014:453012.
10. Raaschou P, Frisell T, Askling J. TNF inhibitor therapy and risk of breast cancer recurrence in patients with rheumatoid arthritis: a nationwide cohort study. Ann Rheum Dis 2015;74:2137–43.
11. Mamtani R, Clark AS, Scott FI, et al. Association between breast cancer recurrence and immunosuppression in rheumatoid arthritis and inflammatory bowel disease. Arthritis Rheum 2016;68:2403–11.
12. Cibere J, Sibley J, Haga M. Rheumatoid arthritis and the risk of malignancy. Arthritis Rheum 1997;40:1580–6.
13. Parekh-Patel A, White RH, Allen M, et al. Risk of cancer among rheumatoid arthritis patients in California. Cancer Causes Control 2009;20:1001–10.
14. Chang SH, Park JK, Lee UJ, et al. Comparison of cancer incidence among patients with rheumatic disease: a retrospective cohort study. Arthritis Res Ther 2014;16:428.
15. Nyberg G, Eriksson O, Westberg NG. Increased incidence of cervical atypia in women with systemic lupus erythematosus treated with chemotherapy. Arthritis Rheum 1981;24:648–50.
16. Blumenfeld Z, Lorber M, Yoffe N, et al. Systemic lupus erythematosus: predisposition for uterine cervical dysplasia. Lupus 1994;3:59–61.
17. Dhar JP, Kmak D, Bhan R, et al. Abnormal cervicovaginal cytology in women with lupus: a retrospective cohort study. Gynecol Oncol 2001;82:4–6.
18. Tam LS, Chan AY, Chan PK, et al. Increased prevalence of squamous intraepithelial lesions in systemic lupus erythematosus: association with human papillomavirus infection. Arthritis Rheum 2004;50:3619–25.

19. Cibere J, Sibley J, Haga M. Systemic lupus erythematosus and the risk of malignancy. Lupus 2001;10:394–400.

20. Liu H, Ding Q, Yang K, et al. Meta-analysis of systemic lupus erythematosus and the risk of cervical neoplasia. Rheumatology (Oxford) 2011;50:343–8.

21. Waisberg MG, Ribeiro AC, Candido WM, et al. Human papillomavirus and chlamydia trachomatis infections in rheumatoid arthritis under anti-TNF therapy: an observational study. Rheumatol Int 2015;35:459–63.

22. Wadstrom H, Frisell T, Sparen P, et al, ARTIS Study Group. Do RA or TNF inhibitors increase the risk of cervical neoplasia or of recurrence of previous neoplasia? A nationwide study from Sweden. Ann Rheum Dis 2016;75:1272–8.

23. Cordtz R, Mellemkjaer L, Glintborg B, et al. Risk of virus-associated cancer in female arthritis patients treated with biological DMARDs-a cohort study. Rheumatology (Oxford) 2016;75:785–6.

24. Kim SC, Schneeweiss S, Liu J, et al. Biologic disease-modifying antirheumatic drugs and risk of high-grade cervical dysplasia and cervical cancer in rheumatoid arthritis: a cohort study. Arthritis Rheumatol 2016;68:2106–13.

25. Bateman H, Yazici Y, Leff L, et al. Increased cervical dysplasia in intravenous cyclophosphamide-treated patients with SLE: a preliminary study. Lupus 2000; 9:542–4.

26. Al-Sherbeni HH, Fahmy AM, Sherif N. Predisposition to cervical atypica in systemic lupus erythematosus: a clinical and cytopathological study. Autoimmune Dis 2015;2015:751853.

27. Tam LS, Chan PK, Ho SC, et al. Natural history of cervical papilloma virus infection in systemic lupus erythematosus - a prospective cohort study. J Rheumatol 2010;37:330–40.

28. Klumb EM, Pinto AC, Jesus GR, et al. Are women with lupus at higher risk of HPV infection? Lupus 2010;19:1485–91.

29. Joura EA, Giuliano AR, Iversen OE, et al. Broad Spectrum HPV Vaccine Study. A 9-valent HPV vaccine against infection and intraepithelial neoplasia in women. N Engl J Med 2015;372:711–23.

30. Petrosky E, Bocchini JA Jr, Hariri S, et al. Use of 9-valent human papillomavirus (HPV) vaccine: updated HPV vaccination recommendations of the advisory committee on immunization practices. MMWR Morb Mortal Wkly Rep 2015;64:300–4.

31. Van Assen S, Agmon-Levin N, Elkayam O, et al. EULAR recommendations for vaccination in adult patients with autoimmune inflammatory rheumatic diseases. Ann Rheum Dis 2011;70:414–22.

32. Mok CC, Ho LY, Fong LS, et al. Immunogenicity and safety of a quadrivalent human papillomavirus vaccine in patients with systemic lupus erythematosus: a case-control study. Ann Rheum Dis 2013;72:659–64.

33. Soybilgic A, Onel KB, Utset T, et al. Safety and immunogenicity of the quadrivalent HPV vaccine in female systemic lupus erythematosus patients aged 12 to 26 years. Pediatr Rheumatol Online J 2013;11:29.

34. Soldevilla HF, Briones SF, Navarra SV. Systemic lupus erythematosus following HPV immunization or infection? Lupus 2012;21:158–61.

35. Ito H, Noda K, Hirai K, et al. A case of systemic lupus erythematosus (SLE) following human papillomavirus (HPV) vaccination. Nihon Rinsho Meneki Gakkai Kaishi 2016;39:145–9.

36. Leval A, Herweijer E, Ploner A, et al. Quadrivalent human papillomavirus vaccine effectiveness: a Swedish national cohort study. J Natl Cancer Inst 2013;105: 469–74.

37. Kim SC, Schneeweiss S, Myers JA, et al. Cancer screening rates in patients with rheumatoid arthritis: no different from the general population. Arthritis Rheumatol 2012;64:3076–82.
38. Quinzanos I, Davis L, Keniston A, et al. Application and feasibility of systemic lupus erythematosus reproductive health care quality indicators at a public urban rheumatology clinic. Lupus 2015;24:203–9.
39. MacLean C, Louie R, Leake B, et al. Quality of care for patients with rheumatoid arthritis. JAMA 2000;28:984–92.
40. Curtis J, Arora T, Narongroeknawin P, et al. The delivery of evidence-based preventive care for older Americans with arthritis. Arthritis Res Ther 2010;12:R144.
41. Kremers H, Bidaut-Russel M, Scott C, et al. Preventive medical services among patients with rheumatoid arthritis. J Rheumatol 2003;30:1940–7.
42. Yazdany J, Tonner C, Trupin L, et al. Provision of preventive health care in systemic lupus erythematosus: data from a large observational cohort study. Arthritis Res Ther 2010;12:R84.
43. Drenkard C, Rask JK, Easley KA, et al. Primary preventive services in patients with systemic lupus erythematosus: Study from a population-based sample in southeast US. Semin Arthritis Rheum 2013;43:209–16.

Contraception in Patients with Rheumatic Disease

Lisa R. Sammaritano, MD

KEYWORDS

- Contraception • Birth control pill • Intrauterine device
- Long-acting reversible contraception • Systemic lupus erythematosus
- Antiphospholipid syndrome

KEY POINTS

- Contraception is an important area of reproductive health for patients with rheumatic diseases given the potential pregnancy risks associated with active disease, teratogenic medications, and severe disease-related damage.
- Long-acting reversible contraceptives, such as intrauterine devices and progestin implants, are most effective and should be encouraged even for nulliparous or adolescent patients who do not have contraindications.
- Antiphospholipid-negative patients with stable systemic lupus erythematosus may use oral combined contraceptives.
- Antiphospholipid-positive patients, or patients with rheumatic disease with other risk factors for thrombosis, should not use estrogen-containing contraceptives.
- Contraceptive methods should be discussed by both the rheumatologist and gynecologist to determine the safest, most effective, and most convenient form for each individual patient.

INTRODUCTION

Counseling patients to plan for pregnancy is an important aspect of care for reproductive-aged patients, especially in the presence of active rheumatic disease, teratogenic medications, or severe disease-related damage. Prepregnancy planning may promote optimal pregnancy outcomes for patients with rheumatic disease, but minimizing unplanned pregnancies relies on the critical assumption that patients use safe and effective contraception. As a result, a basic knowledge of currently available contraceptive methods is essential for both rheumatologists and patients with rheumatic disease.

Effective Contraception

Effectiveness of contraceptive methods varies widely, and counseling for patients must include both the necessity of contraceptive use and also guidance on the safest, most effective methods for that particular patient. Effectiveness is reported

Division of Rheumatology, Hospital for Special Surgery, Weill Cornell Medicine, New York, NY 10021, USA
E-mail address: sammaritanol@hss.edu

Rheum Dis Clin N Am 43 (2017) 173–188
http://dx.doi.org/10.1016/j.rdc.2016.12.001
0889-857X/17/© 2017 Elsevier Inc. All rights reserved.

rheumatic.theclinics.com

in 2 ways: as perfect use (ie, when used exactly as prescribed), and typical use, reflecting real-world use. Perfect use and typical use effectiveness are closest for those methods not directly related to the act of intercourse, and are nearly identical for long-acting reversible contraceptives (LARC) that require no effort on the part of the patient, such as the intrauterine device (IUD) and subdermal implant.[1]

Reversible contraception includes barrier methods, IUDs, and various forms of hormonal contraceptives. Natural or fertility awareness methods are least effective and are not recommended for patients with rheumatic disease for whom unintended pregnancy may have adverse health consequences. Effectiveness rates for commonly used contraceptive methods are summarized in **Table 1**.

LARC methods are clearly most effective: a prospective study of 9256 women showed superior efficacy of LARC (IUD or implant) compared with other contraceptives (including oral contraceptive pills, patch, and vaginal ring). The contraceptive failure rate was 4.55 (per 100 participant-years) for oral, patch, and vaginal ring contraceptives versus 0.27 (per 100 participant-years) for LARC methods.[2] Despite the demonstrated greater efficacy for LARC, the most common contraceptive methods used by women of child-bearing age in the United States are the combined oral contraceptive pill (27%) and female sterilization (28%). Rate of IUD use is about 7%.[3,4]

UNDERUSE OF EFFECTIVE CONTRACEPTION

Effective contraceptive methods are underused by patients with rheumatic disease. In general, patients with rheumatic disease at risk for unplanned pregnancy do not consistently use contraception, and, when they do, they often use a less effective method (usually condoms).

Table 1
Perfect use and typical use effectiveness for contraceptive methods

Method	Effectiveness (%)[a]	
	Perfect Use	Typical Use
None	85	85
Barrier Methods:		
Condom	2	15
Diaphragm	6	16
IUDs:		
Copper IUD	0.6	0.8
LNG-IUD	0.2	0.2
Progesterone Only:		
Progesterone pill	0.5	8
Etonogestrel implant	0.05	0.05
DMPA IM	0.3	3
Combined Hormonal Contraceptives:		
Oral	0.3	9
Transdermal patch	0.3	9
Vaginal ring	0.3	9

Abbreviations: DMPA, depot medroxyprogesterone acetate; IM, intramuscular; LNG, levonorgestrel.
[a] Percentage of women experiencing pregnancy during first year of use.
Adapted from Centers for Disease Control and Prevention (CDC). U.S. medical eligibility criteria for contraceptive use, 2010. MMWR Recomm Rep 2010;59(RR–4):1–86.

Recent survey studies confirm a lower-than-expected rate of contraception use in patients with rheumatic disease.[5,6] One report of contraceptive use among women with systemic lupus erythematosus (SLE) aged 8 to 50 years surveyed 97 women at risk for unplanned pregnancy during the previous 3 months: 55% reported unprotected sex at least once, and 23% reported unprotected sex most of the time.[5] In another study of 86 patients with SLE, 22% reported inconsistent contraceptive use, and 55% used barrier methods. Even more concerning, women on teratogenic medications were no more likely than other women to have used effective contraception.[6] Patients with inflammatory arthritis show similar trends: in another survey, 27% of 94 women at risk for unintended pregnancy who were on the potentially teratogenic drugs methotrexate or leflunomide were not using any form of contraception, although most patients indicated that they were aware of the medications' potential teratogenicity.[7]

Analyses of health care claims databases also show decreased use of effective contraception for women with chronic illnesses, including SLE and rheumatoid arthritis (RA).[8,9] DeNoble and colleagues[8] analyzed prescription contraceptive use for 11,649 women in 1 large health care database, 1869 of whom had a chronic condition, defined as SLE, RA, inflammatory bowel disease, hypertension, asthma, obesity, or hypothyroidism. Over a 3-year period, only 33.5% of women with a chronic condition (vs 41.1% of healthy controls) received prescription contraception (P<.001). Significantly, rates of contraception prescriptions were lowest for the groups with SLE and RA: 21.7% and 20.0% respectively.[8]

Poor use of effective contraception is likely multifactorial. Management of a serious illness may overshadow usual health maintenance issues, and rheumatologists may assume contraceptive counseling is being provided by other physicians. Time allotted for patient visits may also limit discussion. Screening for sexual activity in pediatric rheumatology patients was evaluated in one study of 178 adolescents[10]: rates of screening were low, and physicians reported that limited time was the major barrier, although other factors cited included logistical problems, discomfort with the subject area, and ambivalence about the rheumatologist's role. Other socioeconomic factors may also play a role. Ferguson and colleagues[11] found that one-third of their adult SLE cohort (n = 68) did not receive contraceptive counseling when starting a new medication. Older age, white race, depressive symptoms, and higher SLE disease activity were independently associated with not receiving contraceptive counseling.

TYPES OF CONTRACEPTIVES

Contraceptives vary in terms of effectiveness, but they also vary in terms of availability, convenience of use, and safety. Safety issues are of particular concern for women with rheumatic diseases.

Barrier Contraception

Barrier methods of contraception, most commonly the condom, have significantly lower typical use effectiveness than do hormonal methods or IUDs: 15 out of 100 women using condoms become pregnant during 1 year of use. Despite lower effectiveness, condoms offer the advantages of easy availability and protection against sexually transmitted diseases. Efficacy of barrier contraception is increased if 2 methods are used; for example, condom and spermicide. As a result, this should be a standard recommendation for patients who use barrier protection.[12]

Intrauterine Devices

Although not as commonly used in the United States, the IUD is the most commonly used form of reversible contraception worldwide.[13] IUDs are extremely effective and may be recommended for use even in adolescents and nulliparous women.[14] The most commonly used IUDs contain either copper or the second-generation progesterone levonorgestrel (LNG; 14 or 20 μg/24 h). Copper-containing IUDs remain in place for 10 years, but are often associated with heavier menses and dysmenorrhea. LNG-containing IUDs remain in place for 3 to 5 years. The LNG-IUDs generally reduce dysmenorrhea and menstrual bleeding, with complete amenorrhea in up to 50% of patients by 24 months.[15] The progestin effect of the LNG-IUD is primarily local, although a small proportion of patients report systemic side effects; fertility quickly returns to normal with removal.

Complications associated with IUD use include risk of expulsion (5% over 5 years) and a very low risk of pelvic inflammatory disease (1.6 infections per 1000 women-years) in the 20 days following insertion.[16] Risk of IUD-associated infection in patients on immunosuppressive medications has not been studied, but reports in immunocompromised women infected with HIV show no increased risk of infection.[17] In addition to specific contraindications related to gynecologic disorders, IUD use is discouraged in women at high risk for sexually transmitted diseases; that is, those with multiple sexual partners.

Hormonal Contraception

Hormonal contraceptives include combined estrogen-progesterone and progestin-only preparations. Dose and type of hormone, as well as route of administration, affect both efficacy and risk of side effects.

Combined hormonal contraceptives

The first available birth control pill had 3 to 5 times the estrogen content of current combined oral contraceptives (COCs). Current COCs contain a low dose of synthetic estrogen (ethinyl estradiol or mestranol, 20–50 μg) and a progestin (17-α ethinyl analogues of 19-nortestosterone). The 19-nortestosterones are termed second-generation progestins and include norethindrone and LNG. Third-generation progestins were developed to decrease androgenic side effects and include norgestimate and desogestrel. Drospirenone, an analogue of spironolactone, shows progestational, antiandrogenic, and antimineralocorticoid activity and is considered a fourth-generation progestin.[18] Potential side effects differ according to generation.

Newer formulations of combined (ie, estrogen-progestin) hormonal contraceptives (CHCs) with novel (nonoral) administration methods include the transdermal patch and the intravaginal ring. The transdermal patch is applied weekly for 3 out of 4 weeks, and delivers 20 μg of ethinyl estradiol and 150 μg of norelgestromin every 24 hours. Efficacy is similar to the pill; however, overall estrogen exposure may be increased.[19] The intravaginal ring is kept in place for 3 of 4 weeks and releases 15 μg of ethinyl estradiol and 120 μg of etonogestrel every 24 hours.

Occurrence of serious complications is low and may be limited with careful assessment to exclude patients at greatest risk. Serious complications are usually vascular, including venous thromboembolism (VTE), stroke, and myocardial infarction (MI). There is an increased risk of cervical cancer and a slightly increased risk of breast cancer in current (but not past) users.[18] Effects on the hemostatic system involve multiple mechanisms with an overall net effect that is prothrombotic. The overall risk of VTE in women on current CHCs is increased by a factor of 3 to 5 from the baseline annual risk in healthy women of 1 in 10,000.[20] Nonoral preparations may confer higher risk than do some of the oral preparations.[21]

Both estrogen and progestin contribute to increased VTE risk. Relative risk was increased by a factor of 10 with the earliest COCs, but reducing estrogen content has reduced the risk of oral preparations. At present, variation in type of progestin now accounts for most variability in VTE risk among different CHCs. Third-generation progestins confer greater risk than do second-generation progestins because of greater activated protein C resistance.[22] Relative risks for VTE with selected CHCs are shown in **Table 2**.

CHC-associated risk of VTE is further increased in the presence of genetic or ac-quired thrombophilia, including antiphospholipid antibody (aPL), and is also increased with smoking (>10 cigarettes a day), age greater than 35 years, and obesity (body mass index $\geq$25 kg/m^2).[23] Arterial thrombosis risk is also increased with CHC use. Stroke risk is increased 2-fold and depends on the presence of additional risk factors, including hypertension, migraine, smoking, and older age (>35 years).[24] The likelihood of stroke associated with use of third-generation progestins is no higher than that associated with second-generation progestins, and may be slightly lower.[25] Myocardial infarction risk is also increased, with greatest risk associated with traditional risk factors, including older age, smoking, hypertension, diabetes mellitus, hyperlipidemia, and obesity.[26]

Progestin-only contraceptives

Progestin-only contraceptives (POCs) (including the most effective, LARC) present an alternative option for patients who cannot take estrogen. Oral POCs contain norethindrone or norgestrel: they are less popular than COCs because they have more frequent side effects, particularly irregular vaginal bleeding. It is also important to take the progestin-only pill at the same time each day to ensure stability in serum level.[18]

Other progestin contraceptives confer more stable serum levels through different methods of delivery. Depot medroxyprogesterone acetate (DMPA) is administered as an intramuscular or subcutaneous injection every 3 months. Unlike other progestin methods, it suppresses ovulation. As a result, unlike the progesterone-only pill or LNG-IUD, DMPA may cause reversible bone loss: reduction in bone density in healthy women is 5.7% to 7.5% after 2 years of use.[27] History of fragility fracture, known

Table 2
Risk of venous thromboembolism with selected combined hormonal (estrogen-progestin) contraceptives

Contraceptive	VTE Risk per Year (%)	Adjusted Odds Ratio (95% CI)
No contraception	0.020	1.00
Combined Oral: 30–40 μg Ethinyl Estradiol Plus		
LNG (second generation)	0.055	2.92 (2.23–3.81)
Desogestrel (third generation)	0.099	6.61 (5.60–7.80)
Drospirenone (fourth generation)	0.068	6.37 (5.43–7.47)
Transdermal patch	0.097	7.90 (3.54–17.65)
Vaginal ring	0.078	6.48 (4.69–8.94)

Abbreviation: CI, confidence interval.

Adapted from Stam-Slob MC, Lambalk CB, van de Ree MA. Contraceptive and hormonal treatment options for women with history of venous thromboembolism. BMJ 2015;351:h4847.

osteoporosis, or strong risk factors for osteoporosis (such as corticosteroid use or diagnosis of RA) are generally considered contraindications to use of DMPA. An additional disadvantage is a delayed return to fertility: it is not recommended for patients who plan pregnancy within the next year.

The single-rod etonogestrel subdermal implant is placed in the inner upper arm and releases hormone over a 3-year period. It may inhibit ovulation initially following insertion, but does not consistently inhibit ovulation throughout the 3 years, although other mechanisms remain intact.[18]

Noncontraceptive benefits of POCs are occasionally the primary reason for use and include decreased menstrual bleeding and amelioration of endometriosis symptoms. Minor side effects are common, including irregular breakthrough bleeding (the most common cause of discontinuation) and weight gain. Unpredictable bleeding is greatest within the first 3 months of use and diminishes significantly with time.[18] The risk for thromboembolism with POCs is clearly lower than for CHCs, but the precise degree of risk is debated and is discussed in detail later.[28]

Emergency Contraception

Emergency contraception to prevent pregnancy after unprotected intercourse is widely available. Options include placement of a copper IUD, prescription-only oral selective progesterone receptor modulators (ulipristal or mifepristone), and nonprescription oral LNG. Rheumatic disease, cardiovascular disease, and thrombophilia are not contraindications to the use of emergency contraception.[14]

SPECIFIC ISSUES FOR RHEUMATIC DISEASES

Certain issues are of obvious concern when evaluating the safety of contraceptive methods in patients with rheumatic diseases. Major issues include risk of disease exacerbation, risk of thromboembolism, and potential interaction with medications.

Risk of Disease Exacerbation

Although early uncontrolled reports suggested risk of lupus flare in patients with established disease exposed to COCs, 2 controlled clinical trials published in 2005 did not find a significant increase in risk of flare with COC use in well-defined lupus populations with stable disease activity.[29,30]

The Safety of Estrogen in Lupus Erythematosus National Assessment (SELENA) trial randomized 183 patients with lupus with inactive or stable-active disease to COC (triphasic ethinyl estradiol 35 μg/norethindrone 0.5–1 mg) or placebo for twelve 28-day cycles. Patients with a history of thrombosis or presence of aPL (moderate to high anticardiolipin antibody or positive lupus anticoagulant) were excluded, as were patients with significant disease activity. Severe flare rates at 1 year did not differ (0.084 vs 0.087 for treatment group vs placebo group, respectively). Mild-moderate flares and overall combined flare rates were also equivalent.[29] Sanchez-Guerrero and colleagues[30] compared the use of COC (ethinyl estradiol 30 μg/LNG 150 μg/d) in patients with SLE with 2 alternative contraceptives: an oral POC (LNG 0.3 mg/d) and a copper IUD. Disease activity was similar among the groups, including rates of severe flare, global disease activity, and overall flare. The POC group had a higher rate of discontinuation, and the severe infection rate was slightly higher in the copper IUD group, although there were no instances of pelvic inflammatory disease.[30]

The few studies evaluating lupus activity with POCs do not suggest increased risk of flare.[30] The oral pregnane progestins chlormadinone acetate and cyproterone acetate (antiandrogenic, antiestrogenic weak progestins available in Europe but not the United

States) have been studied as contraceptives in patients with SLE: 187 patients were treated for a mean period of 46 months, there were no thromboses, and a decrease in disease activity was noted.[31]

Use of hormonal contraceptives in rheumatic diseases other than SLE has not generated concern regarding increased disease activity. In contrast, several studies suggest that patients with RA may potentially benefit from treatment with COCs. In one case-control study evaluating 176 women with RA, after adjustments for age, parity, and breastfeeding, the relative risk of developing severe disease with COC use for greater than 5 years was 0.1 (95% confidence interval, 0.01–0.6).[32] Another report of an inception cohort of 132 female patients with RA followed for an average of 12 years suggested a trend for patients using COCs to have both less radiographic joint damage and a better functional level than patients not using COCs.[33] However, a recent systematic review of contraceptive methods in RA did not confirm any effect of hormonal contraceptives on RA progression.[34,35]

Although data regarding risk of disease exacerbation with hormonal contraceptives in patients with rheumatic disease are reassuring, use of CHCs should still be restricted to those patients at low risk. For example, in a United States national sample, 16% of unselected women aged 20 to 51 years were ineligible for COCs based on traditional contraindications.[33] It is to be expected that an even higher proportion of patients with rheumatic disease will be ineligible because of the presence of aPL, active or severe disease, and other usual contraindications.

It is important to keep in mind that the COCs used in the SELENA and Sanchez-Guerrero and colleagues[30] studies were second generation, so absence of flare risk cannot be generalized to those COCs with a higher estrogen content or different administration methods such as the patch or ring (which have not been studied). In addition, the effect of the LNG-IUD, etonogestrel implant or DMPA on disease activity in any rheumatic disease has not been specifically studied, although progestins in general have not been suggested to increase disease activity.

Risk of Thromboembolism

Patients with rheumatic disease are at an increased risk for thrombosis, even those without aPL.[36–39] In one large SLE cohort (n = 1930), risk factors for thrombosis included smoking (odds ratio [OR], 1.25, $P = .011$), longer disease duration (OR, 1.26/5 years; $P = .027 \times 10^{-7}$), nephritis (OR, 1.35, $P = .036$), aPL (OR, 3.22; $P<10^{-9}$), and immunomodulatory medication use (OR, 1.40; $P = .011$).[39] Addition of a CHC increases risk beyond an already increased baseline risk: the OR for VTE risk with CHC use ranges from 2.23 to 6.61 with the same estrogen content, depending on the type and dose of progestin.[21]

Although many rheumatic diseases increase risk of VTE independently of aPL, aPL is probably the most significant risk factor for thrombosis in these patients. Risk seems to be highest for those patients with lupus anticoagulant (LAC) and/or high-titer immunoglobulin G anticardiolipin (aCL).[40] Presence of additional prothrombotic risk factors, including genetic variants such as factor V Leiden or prothrombin gene mutation (G20210A), medical comorbidities such as pregnancy or nephrotic syndrome, or exogenous factors such as bed rest or smoking, additionally increases risk.[41] Prothrombotic genotypes are fairly common and the addition of aPL to other prothrombotic conditions increases the overall risk of thrombosis.[42] Factor V Leiden and the prothrombin gene mutation contribute to risk of VTE in patients with SLE, and risk is potentiated when combined with presence of aPL.[43]

No prospective controlled studies have specifically evaluated the thrombotic risk of CHC use in patients with aPL, for obvious reasons. Case reports describe aPL-positive patients who have developed vascular thrombosis presumably triggered by oral contraceptives.[44] Because aPL increases risk of arterial as well as venous thrombosis, use of CHC almost certainly increases the risk of both types of vascular events in these patients. An increased risk for stroke in presence of aPL and COC use has been shown in the RATIO (Risk of Arterial Thrombosis in Relation to Oral Contraceptives) study, a case-control study evaluating stroke and MI in women less than 50 years of age. The OR for stroke was 43.1 (12.2–152.0) in the presence of LAC, and was further increased to 201.1 (14.5–523.0) in the presence of LAC plus COC.[45] Additional factors that increase the risk of arterial vascular complications in CHC users, such as complicated migraine or atherosclerosis, may be increased in patients with aPL and rheumatic disease, and therefore may further increase risk of stroke or MI.

In the SELENA study, which was designed to assess the risk of lupus flare and not thrombosis, the study design excluded patients with moderate to high aCL titers, any positive LAC, and history of thrombosis. Although some patients in both treatment and placebo groups presumably had low-level aCL (no numbers are reported), there was no increase in thrombotic complications in the COC group versus the placebo group: 2 treated patients and 3 placebo patients developed clots.[29] Treatment with either combined or progestin-only oral contraceptives resulted in similar rates of thrombosis in the Sanchez-Guerrero and colleagues[30] study: 2 patients (of 54) in each group developed VTE (all were reported to be aPL positive).[30]

Use of progestin-only methods is widely accepted as a lower risk method for patients with rheumatic disease unable to use estrogen-containing methods, although degree of risk, if any, is debated. In addition, they may offer a unique advantage in patients with thrombocytopenia or who are on warfarin: they can reduce heavy menstrual blood flow associated with anticoagulation. Several reports describe life-threatening ovarian cyst hemorrhagic rupture in patients with anticoagulated antiphospholipid syndrome (APS) who required surgical hemostasis and blood transfusion; postsurgical treatment with certain progesterone contraceptives was shown to be protective.[46]

The risk of VTE in women using POCs in the general population is not increased. A recent meta-analysis including 8 studies (2 of these with patients at high risk for VTE) showed that POCs overall are not associated with increased risk of VTE compared with nonusers (relative risk [RR] = 1.03; 0.76–1.39). However, in subgroup analysis, the 2 studies that included DMPA (with a small number of patients) did find a significant increased risk of VTE with DMPA (RR = 2.67; 1.29–5.53).[47] This phenomenon has been suggested to be dose related: higher doses of progestins do cause hemostatic activation, and DMPA peak plasma concentrations are 2500 to 7000 pg/mL (compared with 74–166 pg/mL for the LNG-IUD).[48]

In contrast with DMPA, progesterone-only pill VTE risk was not increased in the same meta-analysis (RR = 0.90; 0.57–1.45), nor was risk increased with the LNG-IUD (RR = 0.61, 0.24–1.53)[47] (**Table 3**). Several recent studies focusing on women at increased VTE risk (ie, those with a history of previous VTE) did not identify a higher risk with use of non-DMPA progestin contraceptives.[49–51] There are few data on the etonogestrel subdermal implant thrombosis risk, although thrombosis risk might, in theory, be slightly higher than with LNG-containing preparations because of the inclusion of a third-generation progestin.

Although studies are reassuring and suggest low risk overall, data on patients with rheumatic disease (particularly those with aPL) are limited; as a result, The Centers for Disease Control and Prevention and World Health Organization guidelines for medical eligibility for contraceptive use do not recommend any form of progestin-containing contraception for women with SLE with positive (or unknown) aPL (risk is category 3, "theoretical or proven risks outweigh advantages").[14,52] In contrast, the American

Table 3
Risk of venous thromboembolism with selected progesterone-only contraceptives

Contraceptive	VTE Risk per Year (%)	Adjusted Odds Ratio (95% CI)
No contraception	0.020	1.00
Combined oral: ethinyl estradiol + LNG	0.055	2.92 (2.23–3.81)
Norethisterone (oral) (second generation)	0.014	0.68 (0.30–1.51)
Desogestrel (oral) (third generation)	0.010	0.61 (0.20–1.90)
LNG-IUD (second generation)	0.017	0.61 (0.24–1.53)
Etonogestrel implant (third generation)	0.017	1.40 (0.58–3.38)
DMPA IM (first generation)	NA	2.67 (1.29–5.53)

Abbreviation: NA, not available.
Adapted from Stam-Slob MC, Lambalk CB, van de Ree MA. Contraceptive and hormonal treatment options for women with history of venous thromboembolism. BMJ 2015;351:h4847.

College of Obstetrics and Gynecology (ACOG) guidelines for contraceptive use in women with chronic medical conditions recommend POCs as safer alternatives than estrogen-progestin contraceptives for women with SLE with aPL, active nephritis, and vascular disease.[53]

Despite their increased efficacy, few studies report on the use of LARC methods in patients with rheumatic disease. One case series surveyed 23 anticoagulated aPL patients with LNG-IUDs placed for treatment of menorrhagia associated with anticoagulation: 58.8% of patients reported decreased bleeding, and there were no thromboses.[54]

In summary, POCs are generally safe, and the LNG-IUD and subdermal implant are more effective than estrogen-containing contraceptives. For patients with rheumatic disease, POCs as well as the copper IUD offer more effective alternatives to barrier methods. In particular, the LNG-IUD is an option that seems to be safe for most patients, with no demonstrated increased risk of thrombosis or infection in the general population. DMPA is not a good long-term option for patients with osteoporosis or those on long-term corticosteroid use because of the risk of decrease in bone density. There are no reported data on the etonogestrel subdermal implant in patients with rheumatic disease.

In general, when considering risk of thrombosis in patients with rheumatic disease with contraceptive use, it is advisable to weigh this against VTE risk in the context of pregnancy: the VTE risk in pregnancy and the postpartum period is much higher than that associated with the use of any hormonal contraceptive, including CHCs. Baseline VTE risk in healthy young women is 1 in 10,000 and risk with current COCs is 5 in 10,000. Risk of VTE in pregnancy for healthy young women is 73 in 10,000, for those with a single prothrombotic defect it is 197 in 10,000, and for those with combined prothrombotic defects, it is 776 in 10,000.[55] Therefore, the risks associated with any hormonal contraceptive method must be balanced with the risks of unintended pregnancy.

Medication Interactions

Potential interactions of hormonal contraceptives with other medications may lead to decreased efficacy of either the contraceptive or the alternative medication. Because many patients with rheumatic disease are on multiple medications, it is important to identify potential pharmacologic interactions before recommending CHCs (**Table 4**).

Table 4
Medication interactions with combined hormonal (estrogen-progestin) contraceptives

Medication	Effect with Concomitant CHC	Comments
Antibiotics:		
Penicillins Cephalosporins Macrolides Metronidazole Sulfa Tetracyclines	↓ CHC efficacy	Caused by ↑ intestinal transport and ↓ enterohepatic reabsorption; small effect
Rifampin Griseofulvin Certain antivirals	↓ CHC efficacy	Potentially significant effect
Anticonvulsants:		
Barbiturates Carbamazepine Oxcarbazepine Topiramate	↓ CHC efficacy	
Phenytoin	↑ phenytoin concentration and ↓ CHC efficacy	
Lamotrigine	↓ lamotrigine concentration	
Mycophenolate	Possible ↓ CHC efficacy	
Corticosteroids	↑ steroid concentration	
Cyclosporin	↑ cyclosporine concentration	
Modafinil	↓ CHC efficacy	
Warfarin	↑ or ↓ warfarin effect	
Thyroid hormone	↓ levels of free thyroxine	Caused by ↑ levels of thyroxine-binding globulin
Potassium-sparing diuretics	Hyperkalemia risk with drospirenone-containing CHC	

Data from Fotherby K. Interactions with oral contraceptives. Am J Obstet Gynecol 1990;163:2153–9; and Amy JJ, Tripathi V. Contraception for women: an evidence based overview. Brit Med J 2009;339(7):b2895.

Medications commonly used in patients with rheumatic disease that have potential interactions with estrogen-containing contraceptives include mycophenolate, cyclosporine, corticosteroids, warfarin, anticonvulsants, antivirals, and antiretrovirals.[56,57] Most antibiotics, with the exception of rifampin, do not significantly affect efficacy.[58] Some herbal medications, particularly St John's wort, may also increase clearance of oral contraceptives and decrease efficacy.[59]

SUMMARY

Decisions regarding contraceptive method ultimately depend on the individual patient, her medical condition, and her stage in reproductive life. Summaries of benefits and potential risk are shown in **Tables 5** and **6**. Combined hormonal contraceptives may be used in most patients with rheumatic disease but should not be used in those with active SLE or those at increased risk for thrombosis, including those with history of thrombosis, nephrotic syndrome, positive aPL, or active vasculitis. Progestin-only methods are good alternatives for most patients, and may be useful for decreasing

Table 5
Summary of contraception methods

	Copper IUD	LNG-IUD	Progestin Pill	DMPA	Progestin Implant	COC	Patch	Vaginal Ring
Efficacy (%)[a]	<1	<1	8	3	<1	9	9	9
Convenience	Inserted by MD 10 y	Inserted by MD 3–5 y	Daily oral, same time	Injection by MD, q 3 mo	Inserted by MD 3 y	Daily oral	Apply weekly	Insert monthly
Side effects	Increased cramps/ bleeding	Decreased cramps/ bleeding	Spotting	Decreased bone density Delayed return to fertility	No effect on bone density Rapid return to fertility	Prothrombotic effect Medication interactions		

Abbreviations: MD, physician; q, every.
[a] Typical use efficacy: risk of pregnancy during first year of use.[52]

Table 6
Risks and benefits of contraceptive methods for patients with rheumatic disease

	Copper IUD	LNG-IUD	Progestin Pill	DMPA	Progestin Implant	COC	Patch	Vaginal Ring
Inflammatory arthritis	No data on infection risk in immunocompromised patients with RD, but					May prevent progression to severe disease		Insertion of vaginal ring may be difficult if significant hand or hip arthritis
SLE	no increased risk in other immunodeficiency states. Avoid if multiple sexual partners. No risk of flare		No osteoporosis risk. No risk of flare	Osteoporosis risk: Avoid if risk factors. No risk of flare	No osteoporosis risk. No risk of flare	No increased risk of flare[a]. Avoid drospirenone-containing if renal disease. Avoid if risk factors for thrombosis including aPL (+) nephrotic syndrome, prolonged immobility, surgery	Unknown risk of flare[b] (higher serum estrogen levels than COC)	Unknown risk of flare[b]
aPL positive or APS	No increased thrombotic risk. Increased bleeding	No increased thrombotic risk[c]. Decreased bleeding	No increased thrombotic risk[c]. Decreased bleeding	Possible increased thrombotic risk. Decreased bleeding	Uncertain/low thrombotic risk[b]	Increased risk of thrombosis: avoid		

Abbreviation: RD, rheumatic disease.

[a] No increased risk of flare in stable inactive/mildly active patients with SLE with second-generation COC.

[b] No/limited data.

[c] Degree of risk debated because of lack of studies in APS, but relative risk for high-risk patients (those with history of venous thromboembolism) is not increased.[49-51]

heavy menstrual blood loss in patients on warfarin. Long-acting methods of birth control, such as the IUD, are the most effective contraceptives and are recommended for use in most women. LARCs have the additional benefit of not adding to the daily medication regimen for patients and avoid issues of compliance. Medication interactions may be significant, and should be explored when recommending contraceptives or when starting new rheumatology medications. In addition, when prolonged immobilization is necessary, whether because of disease flare, surgery, or other hospitalization, estrogen-containing contraceptives should be discontinued if possible, and prophylactic heparin therapy added to reduce risk of venous thromboembolism.

Whatever the patient's clinical and social situation, ongoing discussion between the patient, her rheumatologist, and her gynecologist should ensure use of the most appropriate safe, effective, and acceptable contraceptive method.

REFERENCES

1. Amy JJ, Tripathi V. Contraception for women: an evidence based overview. Br Med J 2009;339(7):b2895.
2. Winner B, Peipert JF, Zhao Q, et al. Effectiveness of long-acting reversible contraception. N Engl J Med 2012;366:1998–2007.
3. Jones J, Mosher W, Daniels K. Current contraceptive use in the United States 2006 – 2010, and changes in patterns of use since 1995. Natl Health Stat Report 2012;(60):1–5.
4. Available at: http://www.cdc.gov/nchs/fastats/contraceptive.htm. Accessed August 19, 2016.
5. Schwartz EB, Manzi S. Risk of unintended pregnancy among women with systemic lupus erythematosus. Arthritis Rheum 2008;59(6):863–6.
6. Yazdany J, Trupin L, Kaiser R, et al. Contraceptive counseling and use among women with systemic lupus: a gap in health care quality? Arthritis Care Res 2011;63(3):358–65.
7. Østensen M, Von Esebeck M, Villiger PM. Therapy with immunosuppressive drugs and biological agents and use of contraception in patients with rheumatic disease. J Rheumatol 2007;34(6):1266–9.
8. DeNoble AE, Hall KS, Xu X, et al. Receipt of prescription contraception by commercially insured women with chronic medical conditions. Obstet Gynecol 2014;123(6):1213–20.
9. Champaloux SW, Tepper NK, Curtis KM, et al. Contraceptive use among women with medical conditions in a nationwide privately insured population. Obstetrics Gynecol 2015;126(6):1151–9.
10. Britto MT, Rosenthal SL, Taylor J, et al. Improving rheumatologist' screening for alcohol and sexual activity. Arch Pediatr Adolesc Med 2000;154(5):478–83.
11. Ferguson S, Trupin L, Yazdany J, et al. Who receives contraception counseling when starting new lupus medications? The potential roles of race, ethnicity, disease activity, and quality of communication. Lupus 2016;25(1):12–7.
12. Kestelman P, Trussell J. Efficacy of the simultaneous use of condoms and spermicides. Fam Plann Perspect 1991;23:226–7.
13. D'Arcangues C. Worldwide use of intrauterine devices for contraception. Contraception 2007;75(6):S2–7.
14. World Health Organization. Medical eligibility for criteria for contraceptive use. 2015. Available at: http://apps.who.int/iris/bitstream/10665/181468/1/9789241549158_eng.pdf. Accessed August 19, 2016.

15. Hidalgo M, Bahamondes L, Perrotti M, et al. Bleeding patterns and clinical performance of the levonorgestrel-releasing intrauterine system (Mirena) up to two years. Contraception 2002;65(2):129–32.
16. Lyus R, Lohr P, Prager S. Use of the Mirena LNG-IUS and Paragard CuT380A intrauterine devices in nulliparous women. Contraception 2010;81(5):367–71.
17. Stringer EM, Kaseba C, Levy J, et al. A randomized trial of the intrauterine device versus hormonal contraception in women who are infected with the human immunodeficiency virus. Am J Obstet Gynecol 2007;197(2):144.e1-8.
18. Rivlin C, Westhoff C. Family planning. In: Lobo RA, Gershenson DM, Lentz GM, et al, editors. Comprehensive Gynecology. Philadelphia: Elsevier Mosby; 2016. p. 237–57.
19. Burkman RT. Transdermal hormonal contraception: benefits and risks. Am J Obstet Gynecol 2007;197(2):134.e1-6.
20. Martinelli I. Risk factors in venous thromboembolism. Thromb Haemost 2001;86: 395–403.
21. Stam-Slob MC, Lambalk CB, van de Ree MA. Contraceptive and hormonal treatment options for women with history of venous thromboembolism. BMJ 2015;351: h4847.
22. Van Hylckama Vlieg A, Helmerhorst FM, Vandenbroucke JP, et al. The venous thromboembolic risk of oral contraceptives, effects of oestrogen dose and progestin type: results of the MEGA case-control study. Br Med J 2009;339:b2921.
23. Tanis BC, Rosendaal FR. Venous and arterial thrombosis during oral contraceptive use: risks and risk factors. Semin Vasc Med 2003;3(1):69–84.
24. Kemmeren JM, Tanis BC, van den Bosch MA, et al. Risk of Arterial Thrombosis in Relation to Oral Contraceptives (RATIO) study: oral contraceptives and the risk of ischemic stroke. Stroke 2002;33:1202–8.
25. Lidegaard Ø, Løkkegaard E, Jensen A, et al. Thrombotic stroke and myocardial infarction with hormonal contraception. N Engl J Med 2012;366:2257–66.
26. Lewis MA, Heinnemann LAJ, Spitzer WO, et al. The use of oral contraceptives and the occurrence of acute myocardial infarction in young women. Results from the Transnational Study on Oral Contraceptives and the Health of Young Women. Contraception 1997;56:129–40.
27. American College of Obstetricians and Gynecologists Committee on Gynecologic Practice. ACOG Comm Opinion number 415: Depo-medroxyprogesterone acetate and bone effects. Obstet Gynecol 2008;12:727–30.
28. Hennessy S, Berlin JA, Kinman JL, et al. Risk of venous thromboembolism from oral contraceptives containing gestodene and desogestrel versus levonorgestrel: a meta-analysis and formal sensitivity analysis. Contraception 2001;64:125–33.
29. Petri M, Kim MY, Kalunian KC, et al. Combined oral contraceptives in women with systemic lupus erythematosus. N Engl J Med 2005;353:2550–8.
30. Sanchez-Guerrero J, Uribe AG, Jimenez-Santana L, et al. A trial of contraceptive methods in women with systemic lupus erythematosus. N Engl J Med 2005;353: 2539–49.
31. Chabbert-Buffet N, Amoura Z, Scarabin PY, et al. Pregnane progestin contraception in systemic lupus erythematosus: a longitudinal study of 187 patients. Contraception 2011;83(3):229–37.
32. Jorgensen C, Picot MC, Bologna C, et al. Oral contraception, parity, breast feeding, and severity of rheumatoid arthritis. Ann Rheum Dis 1996;55(2):94–8.
33. Drossaers-Bakker KW, Zwinderman AH, Van Zeben D, et al. Pregnancy and oral contraceptive use do not significantly influence outcome in long term rheumatoid arthritis. Ann Rheum Dis 2002;61(5):405–8.

34. Farr SL, Folger SG, Paulsen ME, et al. Safety of contraceptive methods for women with rheumatoid arthritis: a systematic review. Contraception 2010;82(1):64–71.
35. Shortridge E, Miller K. Contraindications to oral contraceptive use among women in the United States 1999-2001. Contraception 2007;75:355–60.
36. Chung WS, Peng CL, Lin CL, et al. Rheumatoid arthritis increases the risk of deep vein thrombosis and pulmonary thromboembolism: a nationwide cohort study. Ann Rheum Dis 2014;73(10):1774–80.
37. Chung WS, Lin CL, Sung FC, et al. Increased risks of deep vein thrombosis and pulmonary embolism in Sjögren syndrome: a nationwide cohort study. J Rheumatol 2014;41(5):909–15.
38. Gaffo AL. Thrombosis in vasculitis. Best Pract Res Clin Rheumatol 2013;27(1): 57–67.
39. Kaiser R, Cleveland CM, Criswell LA. Risk and protective factors for thrombosis in systemic lupus erythematosus: results from a large, multi-ethnic cohort. Ann Rheum Dis 2009;68(2):238–41.
40. Danowski A, de Azevedo MNL, Petrie M. Determinants of risk for venous and arterial thrombosis in primary antiphospholipid syndrome and in antiphospholipid syndrome with systemic lupus erythematosus. J Rheumatol 2009;36(6):1195–9.
41. Erkan D, Harrison MJ, Levy R, et al. Aspirin for primary thrombosis prevention in the antiphospholipid syndrome: a randomized, double-blind, placebo-controlled trial in asymptomatic antiphospholipid antibody–positive individuals. Arthritis Rheum 2007;56(7):2382–91.
42. Forastiero R, Martinuzzo M, Adamczuk Y, et al. The combination of thrombophilic genotypes is associated with definite antiphospholipid syndrome. Haematologica 2001;86(7):735–41.
43. Brouwer JL, Bijl M, Veeger NJ, et al. The contribution of inherited and acquired thrombophilic defects, alone or combined with antiphospholipid antibodies, to venous and arterial thromboembolism in patients with systemic lupus erythematosus. Blood 2004;104:143–8.
44. Girolami A, Zanon E, Zanardi S, et al. Thromboembolic disease developing during oral contraceptive therapy in young females with antiphospholipid antibodies. Blood Coagul Fibrinolysis 1996;7:497–501.
45. Urbanus RT, Siegerink B, Roest M, et al. Antiphospholipid antibodies and risk of myocardial infarction and ischaemic stroke in young women in the RATIO study: a case-control study. Lancet Neurol 2009;8(11):998–1005.
46. Yamakami LYS, de Araujo DB, Silva CA, et al. Severe hemorrhagic corpus luteum complicating anticoagulation in antiphospholipid syndrome. Lupus 2011;20: 523–6.
47. Mantha S, Karp R, Raghavan V, et al. Assessing the risk of venous thromboembolic events in women taking progestin-only contraception: a meta-analysis. BMJ 2012;345:e4944.
48. Rott H. Thrombotic risks of oral contraceptives. Curr Opin Obstet Gynecol 2012; 24:235–40.
49. Conard J, Plu-Bureau G, Bahi N, et al. Progestogen-only contraception in women at high risk of venous thromboembolism. Contraception 2004;70(6):437–41.
50. Vaillant-Roussel H, Ouchchane L, Dauphin C, et al. Risk factors for recurrence of venous thromboembolism associated with the use of oral contraceptives. Contraception 2011;84(5):e23–30.
51. Le Moigne E, Tromeur C, Delluc A, et al. Risk of recurrent venous thromboembolism on progestin-only contraception: cohort study. Haematologica 2016;101(1): e12–4.

52. Centers for Disease Control and Prevention (CDC). U.S. medical eligibility criteria for contraceptive use, 2010. MMWR Recomm Rep 2010;59(RR-4):1–86.
53. ACOG Committee on Practice Bulletins – Gynecology. ACOG practice bulletin number 73: use of hormonal contraception in women with coexisting medical conditions. Obstet Gynecol 2006;107:1453–72.
54. Pisoni CN, Cuadrado MJ, Khamashta MA, et al. Treatment of menorrhagia associated with oral anticoagulation: efficacy and safety of the levonorgestrel releasing intrauterine device (Mirena coil). Lupus 2006;15(12):877–80.
55. van Vlijmen EF, Veeger NJ, Middeldorp S, et al. Thrombotic risk during oral contraceptive use and pregnancy in women with factor V Leiden or prothrombin mutation: a rational approach to contraception. Blood 2011;118(8):2055–61.
56. Fotherby K. Interactions with oral contraceptives. Am J Obstet Gynecol 1990;163:2153–9.
57. Sievers TM, Rossi SJ, Ghobrial RM, et al. Mycophenolate mofetil. Pharmacotherapy 1997;17(6):1178–97.
58. Dickinson BD, Altman R, Nielsen N, et al. Drug interactions between oral contraceptives and antibiotics. Obstet Gynecol 2001;98(5):853–60.
59. Hall SD, Wang Z, Huang SM, et al. The interaction between St. John's wort and an oral contraceptive. Clin Pharmacol Ther 2003;74:525–35.

Preconception Counseling

Monika Østensen, MD*

KEYWORDS

- Rheumatic disease • Pregnancy • Risk assessment • Communication

KEY POINTS

- Address family planning in all patients of fertile age. Physicians should actively offer information on reproduction issues to all patients, even those who do not specifically ask.
- Ideal conditions for pregnancy are: conception at a stage of remission or minimal disease activity while on stable, pregnancy-compatible medication.
- Address medication concerns and the benefits of optimal disease control in pregnancy with all patients.
- Points discussed during preconception counseling should be shared with all doctors and health professionals involved in the care of a pregnant patient.

INTRODUCTION

Given that rheumatic diseases (RDs) have frequent onset during the reproductive years as well as a female predominance, discussion of reproduction issues with patients of fertile age is an important issue. Patients often have significant information needs when it comes to meeting the challenges related to pregnancy and parenting.[1] When a patient brings up a desire for children, most rheumatologists offer preconception counseling based on clinical and laboratory assessment of the disease. The aims of counseling are to assist in planning a pregnancy and to optimize management before and throughout pregnancy. Doctors and health professionals engaging in counseling have specific goals in mind; in addition, the patient herself has special needs that must be met if counseling fulfills its intention: to secure a good pregnancy outcome for mother and child.

Information on family planning not only should be given to patients who ask for it but also actively offered to adolescent patients, to patients who are not in a relationship, and also to those who already have children provided they are aged 18 to 45 years. Partners not present at a first consultation may appear at a later point, and new

Disclosure Statement: The author has nothing to disclose.
National Advisory Unit on Pregnancy and Rheumatic Diseases, Department of Rheumatology, Trondheim University Hospital, Trondheim, Norway
* Olav Kyrres Gate 13, N 7006 Trondheim, Norway.
E-mail address: monika.ostensen@gmail.com

relationships may develop over time, so that patients may desire children with a new partner even when they already have children from a previous relationship.

FERTILITY

Fertility issues should be discussed when a patient plans a pregnancy, particularly before withdrawal of effective therapy that has kept the patient in remission. Discontinuation of effective medications when pregnancy is planned may result in a flare, especially when the patient fails to conceive over a prolonged period of time.[2] Frequent monitoring after drug withdrawal and initiation of alternative therapy compatible with pregnancy are, therefore, required. Should a patient fail to conceive after more than 6 months, referral to a gynecologist and investigation of fertility of the couple is advisable (see Emily C Somers and Wendy Marder's article, "Infertility – Prevention and Management," in this issue).

CONTRACEPTION

A major point of addressing family planning in all patients of fertile age is to avoid unplanned pregnancies and the maternal and fetal risks connected with it. Counseling on and regular practice of effective birth control is the only way to prevent unplanned pregnancy.[3] It is the responsibility of the treating rheumatologist to address contraception actively in all patients at risk for unplanned pregnancy (see Lisa R. Sammaritano's article, "Contraception in Rheumatic Disease Patients," in this issue). No prescription for methotrexate, mycophenolate mofetil, cyclophosphamide, or other teratogenic medication should be given without first excluding pregnancy and ensuring comprehensive information on safe and effective birth control. Patients with active disease and a desire for children should practice effective birth control until the disease has improved or has gone into remission for at least 6 months.

THE COURSE OF RHEUMATIC DISEASE IN PREGNANCY

The type of RD influences both the effect of pregnancy on disease symptoms and the impact of the chronic disease on pregnancy (**Table 1**). Rheumatoid arthritis (RA) and other polyarticular RDs like polyarticular juvenile idiopathic arthritis (JIA) improve spontaneously during pregnancy in a major proportion of pregnant patients.[4] Axial arthritis either does not change or is aggravated during pregnancy.[5] Systemic lupus erythematosus (SLE) flares in up to 50% of pregnancies, including major organ involvement in up to 25%.[5]

The impact of RD on pregnancy largely relates to the extent of inflammation present. A disease where arthritis in peripheral joints is the predominant symptom, with no or few organ manifestations and with no or few autoantibodies, tends not to impair the course of pregnancy to a major extent. In contrast, multiorgan involvement or the presence of certain autoantibodies, as in antiphospholipid syndrome (APS), can result in several pregnancy complications with harmful effects both in mother and fetus.[4] Internal organ involvement, such as in SLE or in antineutrophil cytoplasmic autoantibody–positive small vessel vasculitis, predisposes to increased risk of various pregnancy complications (see **Table 1**).

RISK ASSESSMENT

Risk assessment for possible maternal or fetal risks during a future pregnancy is essential for counseling an individual patient and adjusting therapy.[6] Disease activity should be assessed by standard criteria. A clinical and laboratory work-up should be

Table 1
Maternal and fetal risks in rheumatic diseases during pregnancy

Disease	Most Frequent Maternal Risks	Fetal Risks	Major Points of Counseling
Diseases with peripheral arthritis as major symptom			
RA	Active RA in 10%–25% of pregnancies	Prematurity and lower birthweight with active maternal disease	In patients in remission, low to moderate risk Continue therapy that supports remission.
Spondyloarthropathies	Active disease in approximately 50% of pregnancies	Prematurity and lower birthweight with active maternal disease	Low to moderate risk, but need to control pain, stiffness, and impaired function in spine and joints
JIA	Active disease most prevalent in systemic JIA	Prematurity and lower birthweight with active maternal disease	In patients in remission, low to moderate risk Continue therapy that supports remission, particularly in systemic JIA.
Diseases with systemic involvement (skin, muscles, internal organs, and arthritis)			
SLE	Flare during pregnancy in 35%–70% of patients, development of hypertension and preeclampsia, premature delivery	Fetal loss, intrauterine growth restriction, prematurity, low birthweight, neonatal lupus syndromes	High risk, follow-up by experts; continue immunosuppressive medications compatible with pregnancy.
Systemic sclerosis	Flares not more frequent than outside pregnancy	Prematurity	High risk with early stage disease and with organ involvement
Dermatomyositis/polymyositis	Flare rate not studied	Prematurity and lower birthweight with active maternal disease	High risk, needs follow-up by interdisciplinary team; refer to tertiary center.
Vasculitis	If in remission, slightly increased risk for flare. Development of hypertension and preeclampsia, premature delivery	Fetal loss, intrauterine growth restriction, prematurity, low birthweight	High risk, needs follow-up by interdisciplinary team; refer to tertiary center.
APS	Thrombosis, preeclampsia, HELLP syndrome	Fetal loss, intrauterine growth restriction, prematurity, low birthweight	High risk for obstetric complications and thrombosis; follow-up by experts; anticoagulation throughout pregnancy

performed and potential risk factors for pregnancy complications should be identified, including Sjögren antibodies (anti-Ro/SSA and anti-La/SSB) and antiphospholipid antibodies (aPLs).[7] The work-up allows stratification into a high-risk, moderate-risk, or low-risk profile (**Table 2**). A high-risk profile suggests a substantial risk to the health of mother and/or fetus in pregnancy.

Patients Who Should Postpone Pregnancy

Certain patients should be counseled to postpone pregnancy, among them women with new-onset RD. At an early stage of disease, the pattern of disease severity is not yet apparent and frequent changes in drug treatment are often necessary. A patient with early RD or with active disease should postpone pregnancy until remission or stable disease is achieved and has persisted for at least 6 months.[7] This strategy, however, must be balanced against the disadvantages that advanced maternal age can exert on fertility and pregnancy outcome.[8] In countries where most women are educated and pursue a career, maternal age at a first pregnancy has increased to above 30 years of age. For a patient in her fourth decade who desires children, it seems prudent not to delay pregnancy indefinitely.

Some conditions may seriously threaten maternal and fetal/neonatal health. Patients with severe pulmonary or cardiac involvement, including symptomatic pulmonary hypertension, extensive restrictive lung disease, and cardiomyopathy, as well as women with previous hemolysis, elevated liver enzymes, and low platelet count occurring in association with preeclampsia (HELLP) syndrome should be discouraged from pregnancy because of increased morbidity and mortality.[7,9] Patients with recent arterial thrombosis or current active renal disease should likewise postpone pregnancy.[6]

Maternal Risks in Pregnancy

A major maternal risk for the mother is a flare during pregnancy[5]; however, the propensity for a flare and the flare rate differ among the RDs and depend on type of disease (see **Table 1**). Women with current or recent activity at the time of conception and those who withdraw effective therapy are more likely to suffer a disease flare regardless of diagnosis.[10–13] A flare reduces daily activities, requires escalation of therapy, and increases the risk of pregnancy complications.

Table 2
Stratification of a patient planning pregnancy or currently pregnant into low risk, moderate risk, and high risk before/during pregnancy

Low Risk	Moderate Risk	High Risk
Disease in remission or stable, low disease activity	Disease in remission or stable, low disease activity	Active disease, organ involvement, or organ damage
No aPLs or anti-Ro/SS-A antibodies	No teratogenic drugs but harmful lifestyle factors or comorbidities present	Presence of aPLs or anti-Ro/SS-A antibodies
No comorbidities[a]		Presence of comorbidities and/or harmful lifestyle factors; active disease and therapy with teratogenic drugs
No teratogenic drugs		
No harmful lifestyle factors[b]		

[a] Comorbidities: hypertension, chronic renal disease, endocrine disease, and obesity.
[b] Lifestyle factors: nicotine, alcohol, and recreational drugs.

Several RDs show an increased incidence of preeclampsia, among them SLE, APS, and small vessel vasculitis.[14] Renal disease and/or chronic hypertension increases the risk of developing preeclampsia.[15] Preeclampsia is a failure of proper placenta development, promoted by a proinflammatory environment.[4] In general, patients with no or few organ manifestations, no comorbidities, and without aPLs have little to no increased risk for the development of preeclampsia.

Several population-based studies from different geographic areas have found a 1.5 to 2.0 increased risk for caesarean section (CS) in patients with RD.[16,17] In most studies, no distinction has been made between acute and elective CS. A Norwegian population-based study, including patients with inflammatory arthritides, examined both acute CS and elective CS separately.[18] Acute CS was not observed more often in RD patients than in healthy pregnant women.[18] An elective CS may be related to patient desire or the choice of an obstetrician who may anticipate problems during delivery. Except for presence of obstetric complications, however, vaginal delivery is possible and should be encouraged for most patients.

Women with RD are sometimes concerned about the outcome of a subsequent pregnancy, particularly in the presence of a previous adverse pregnancy outcome.[19] Several studies have shown that adverse outcomes are more frequently encountered in first births,[20,21] possibly because of less awareness or monitoring in patients with new onset disease. The disease course in one pregnancy does not, however, usually predict the course in a subsequent pregnancy, as shown in patients with RA.[22]

Fetal Risks in Pregnancy

Patients with RD planning a pregnancy should be informed about the increased risk of adverse fetal outcomes in a manner that, although not alarming, is clear and straightforward to encourage adherence to frequent monitoring and necessary therapy. They likewise should understand that although optimal therapy can reduce pregnancy complications and adverse outcomes, it cannot guarantee their complete prevention.

Pregnancies in women with RD are characterized by an increased incidence of fetal loss, prematurity, and intrauterine growth restriction.[4,23] A population-based study of SLE pregnancies showed an increased risk of prematurity as well as perinatal deaths.[24] Active lupus nephritis, previous history of fetal death, and the presence of aPLs have been shown predictive factors for fetal loss in lupus pregnancies.[25–27] Another study of 265 SLE pregnancies found that active SLE in the 3 months prior to conception corresponded with a 4-fold increase in pregnancy loss.[25] A population-based study from the Medical Birth Registry of Norway found a higher risk of both early (before gestational week 12) and late (week 12–22) miscarriage in women with RA[28]; however, other smaller studies have not reported an increased miscarriage rate in RA.[29]

Preterm birth (delivery at less than 37 weeks of gestation) is one of the most common adverse outcomes of pregnancies in women with RD.[23,30] Risk factors that predict premature delivery include active disease at conception and in the first trimester.[12,13,25] A prospective cohort study in 440 women with RA found that preterm delivery and small-for-gestational-age infants were associated with increasing disease severity.[13] Other predictors for prematurity in RD are use of greater than 10 mg of prednisone daily, renal disease, aPLs, hypertension, preeclampsia, premature rupture of membranes, and fetal compromise.[7,13,15,26] The same factors increase the risk of intrauterine growth restriction and small-for-gestational-age infants.[23]

Low birthweight has been associated with high disease activity and immunosuppressive therapy.[13] Preterm delivery and infants of lower birthweight have been reported in RA women with high disease activity or on therapy with prednisone.[13,31] Two prospective studies comprising 285 RA pregnancies found birthweight within normal range but lower than in healthy women and even lower in infants of RA mothers with high disease activity.[31,32]

The differences observed in the rate of adverse pregnancy outcomes reported from different countries are likely multifactorial and influenced by the type of health care available, access to methods of contraception, availability of high-risk pregnancy units, and coverage of costs by insurance companies or governmental institutions. Neonatal outcomes depend to a great extent on the quality of prenatal care. Access to optimal health care may not be available for patients living in rural areas or patients of low socioeconomic status; therefore, a substantial risk for adverse pregnancy outcomes remains for a large proportion of patients.

Autoantibodies as Risk Factors

Certain autoantibodies can exert harmful effects on the outcome of pregnancy or on the fetus. Maternal anti-Ro/SSA and anti-La/SSB antibodies are present in women with SLE, Sjögren syndrome, and other autoimmune diseases, and asymptomatic carriers cross the placenta and can cause neonatal lupus syndrome (see Pascal H.P. de Jong1 and Radboud J.E.M. Dolhain's article, "Fertility, Pregnancy and Lactation in Rheumatoid Arthritis," in this issue). Skin rashes, thrombocytopenia, and elevated liver enzymes are transient forms of neonatal lupus syndrome. The most serious presentation is congenital heart block, a rare condition occurring in approximately 2% of primigravidae carriers of anti-Ro/SSA and anti-La/SSB antibodies. Appropriate prepregnancy counseling by a health care provider with specific knowledge who can give relevant and understandable information is essential and may reduce undue anxiety regarding risk in anti-Ro/SSA and anti-La/SSB antibody-positive women.[33]

Presence of significant and persistently positive titers of aPLs increases the risk for adverse pregnancy outcomes, including unexplained spontaneous abortions before 10 weeks of gestation, intrauterine fetal death, and 1 or more premature births of a morphologically normal neonate before 34 weeks of gestation.[34] Women with aPLs are in general at a higher risk for hypertension, preeclampsia, fetal death, placental insufficiency with growth restriction, and prematurity.[35–37] Several studies have identified combined positivity for lupus anticoagulant, anticardiolipin antibodies, and anti–β_2-glycoprotein I as a significant risk factor.[36,37] Women with consistent moderate to high levels of aPL or the presence of APS must be counseled regarding the overall higher risk of thrombosis, pregnancy loss, and preeclampsia as well as the potential need for anticoagulation during pregnancy and the postpartum period.[7] Whether asymptomatic carriers of aPLs are at an increased risk of pregnancy complications or thrombosis is a matter of debate.[7]

RA patients positive for rheumatoid factor or antibodies to citrullinated protein antigens (ACPAs) and those with currently active disease have significantly less chance for spontaneous improvement in disease during pregnancy and are at higher risk for adverse outcomes. RA patients without rheumatoid factor or ACPAs and those with low disease activity or in remission are the most likely to remain inactive during pregnancy.[38]

ADJUSTMENT OF DRUG THERAPY

Women who plan a pregnancy often stop taking medications out of fear of fetal harm, especially in the first trimester. Abrupt withdrawal of all drugs when a pregnancy is planned, however, may result in a flare with undue suffering for the patient and risk for the pregnancy. Unfortunately, a considerable gap exists between the view of the physician and the understanding of the patient regarding the benefit of drug treatment.[39,40] A discussion of the why and when of all patient medications, not only teratogenic drugs, is of utmost importance at preconception counseling. Uncertainty in regard to which drugs are compatible with pregnancy can result in ill-advised medication withdrawal or even in termination of pregnancy. For example, a higher rate of induced abortions in RA patients treated with tumor necrosis factor (TNF) inhibitors than in patients not receiving these agents was found in 1 study.[41] In contrast, patients treated with methotrexate had lower rates of induced abortions than unexposed patients.[41] Women treated with TNF inhibitors may have been misinformed about the fetal risk and choose termination out of fear of harm to their child.

An increasing proportion of pregnant women search the Internet for information on drugs during pregnancy,[39] which may lead to misinterpretation of data, creating undue anxiety. It is prudent to ask patients what information they have already received either through social media, from other patients or family, or from other health professionals involved in their care. Misunderstandings and concerns can then be evaluated and clarified.

DECISION SHARING BETWEEN THE PATIENT AND SPECIALISTS

Patients who are pregnant meet several different medical specialists; with multiple specialists, however, comes a risk that different physicians give conflicting advice on medications in pregnancy.[39] Often patients listen to the most restrictive advice out of fear of harm to their baby. Therefore, it is important to inform patients about not only the risk but also the benefit of medications. Two recent studies have analyzed published data on antirheumatic drugs in pregnancy and lactation.[42,43] The recommendations of these studies can guide a clinician toward appropriate use of medications in pregnancy and lactation based on the most recent data and analyses. Providing as much information as possible helps patients understand that effective disease control during pregnancy is important for a normal pregnancy course and for fetal and neonatal health. Patients should be counseled about the importance of controlling a flare of disease during pregnancy, even when short-term high-dose corticosteroids or drugs not approved for pregnancy are necessary. In addition, first-line, second-line, and even third-line options for effective drug therapy should be offered along with a clear discussion of potential risks and benefits for each. Presenting the full range of options to pregnant women enables patients to make their own decisions regarding medication during pregnancy.

Pregnant women may have pain, fever, or infections during pregnancy and may treat themselves with over-the-counter (OTC) drugs. OTC medications must, therefore, be discussed with patients. Pregnant women are often not aware that OTC drugs and multisubstance pain medications contain nonsteroidal anti-inflammatory drugs (NSAIDs) or paracetamol and codeine that may add to or interact with their established antirheumatic pharmacotherapy. Without this knowledge, they may ingest high doses of NSAIDs that can cause serious side effects, particularly in late pregnancy.[44]

It is useful to address breastfeeding and the probability of relapse of RD during the postpartum period early on with patients so they are aware of this potential risk and ideally have a plan in place for therapy should this occur. Patients should be encouraged to seek help immediately when a flare occurs and not to avoid all therapy out of fear of harming the breastfed infant. Many drugs are compatible with lactation.[42,43]

MONITORING DURING PREGNANCY

Type and frequency of pregnancy monitoring should be agreed on with patients at the outset, and communication established between the rheumatologist, patient, and other health care providers involved in follow-up. Good collaboration during pregnancy by a specialist team that includes a rheumatologist/specialist in internal medicine, obstetrician, and specialist in fetal medicine increases the chance for a successful pregnancy, even for RD with organ involvement. The type and frequency of monitoring depends on the severity of an individual's disease as well as the maternal and fetal risk factors present at conception.

GENERAL RECOMMENDATIONS

Lifestyle adjustments before pregnancy include discontinuation of smoking, using no alcohol or recreational drugs during pregnancy, and maintaining a healthy diet that contains multiple vitamins. Obese women should be encouraged to lose weight before pregnancy.[45] Importance of folic acid supplementation during the early stages of pregnancy needs to be emphasized,[46] particularly in patients who have received therapy with methotrexate or are treated with sulfasalazine.

SUMMARY

A multinational survey study on family planning and pregnancy issues for female patients of childbearing age has shown that medical specialists often fail to give adequate information and support to women with chronic inflammatory diseases.[39] A major problem was a lack of communication between specialists, resulting in inconsistent advice and information. A well-functioning and open route of communication between health professionals engaged in the care of an individual patient is particularly important when counseling a patient about the timing of and therapy during a pregnancy. Finally, the likelihood of good maternal and child outcomes is best when patients are well informed and actively engaged in decision making before conception, during pregnancy, and in the postpartum period.

REFERENCES

1. Ackerman IN, Briggs AM, Ngian GS, et al. Closing the pregnancy-related information gap for women with rheumatoid arthritis: more can be done to support women and their families. Rheumatology 2016;55:1343–4.
2. Jawaheer D, Zhu JL, Nohr EA, et al. Time to pregnancy among women with rheumatoid arthritis. Arthritis Rheum 2011;63:1517–21.
3. Ostensen M. Connective tissue diseases: contraception counseling in SLE – an often forgotten duty? Nat Rev Rheumatol 2011;7:315–6.
4. Østensen M, Cetin I. Autoimmune connective tissue diseases. Best Pract Res Clin Obstet Gynaecol 2015;29:658–70.
5. Østensen M, Villiger PM, Förger F. Interaction of pregnancy and autoimmune rheumatic disease. Autoimmun Rev 2012;11:A437–46.
6. Ruiz-Irastorza G, Khamashta MA. Lupus and pregnancy: integrating clues from the bench and bedside. Eur J Clin Invest 2011;41:672e8.
7. Soh MC, Nelson-Piercy C. High-risk pregnancy and the rheumatologist. Rheumatology (Oxford) 2015;54:572–87.
8. Khalil A, Syngelaki A, Maiz N, et al. Maternal age and adverse pregnancy outcome: a cohort study. Ultrasound Obstet Gynecol 2013;42:634–43.
9. Chakravarty EF, Khanna D, Chung L. Pregnancy outcomes in systemic sclerosis, primary pulmonary hypertension, and sickle cell disease. Obstet Gynecol 2008; 111(4):927–34.

10. Stojan G, Baer AN. Flares of systemic lupus erythematosus during pregnancy and the puerperium: prevention, diagnosis and management. Expert Rev Clin Immunol 2012;8(5):439–53.

11. Koh JH, Ko HS, Kwok SK, et al. Hydroxychloroquine and pregnancy on lupus flares in Korean patients with systemic lupus erythematosus. Lupus 2015;24:210–7.

12. Langen ES, Chakravarty EF, Liaquat M, et al. High rate of preterm birth in pregnancies complicated by rheumatoid arthritis. Am J Perinatol 2014;31:9–14.

13. Bharti B, Lee SE, Lindsay SP, et al. Disease severity and pregnancy outcomes in women with rheumatoid arthritis: results from the organization of teratology information specialists autoimmune diseases in pregnancy project. J Rheumatol 2015;42:1376–82.

14. Spinillo A, Beneventi F, Locatelli E, et al. Early, incomplete, or preclinical autoimmune systemic rheumatic diseases and pregnancy outcome. Arthritis Rheum 2016. http://dx.doi.org/10.1002/art.39737.

15. Bramham K, Hunt BJ, Bewley S, et al. Pregnancy outcomes in systemic lupus erythematosus with and without previous nephritis. J Rheumatol 2011;38:1906–13.

16. Nørgaard M, Larsson H, Pedersen L, et al. Rheumatoid arthritis and birth outcomes: a Danish and Swedish nationwide prevalence study. J Intern Med 2010;268:329–37.

17. Barnabe C, Faris PD, Quan H. Canadian pregnancy outcomes in rheumatoid arthritis and systemic lupus erythematosus. Int J Rheumatol 2011;2011:345727.

18. Wallenius M, Skomsvoll JF, Irgens LM, et al. Pregnancy and delivery in women with chronic inflammatory arthritides with a specific focus on first birth. Arthritis Rheum 2011;63(6):1534–42.

19. Shand AW, Algert CS, March L, et al. Second pregnancy outcomes for women with systemic lupus erythematosus. Ann Rheum Dis 2013;72(4):547–51.

20. Wallenius M, Salvesen KÅ, Daltveit AK, et al. Rheumatoid arthritis and outcomes in first and subsequent births based on data from a national birth registry. Acta Obstet Gynecol Scand 2014;93:302–7.

21. Saavedra MA, Sánchez A, Morales S, et al. Primigravida is associated with flare in women with systemic lupus erythematosus. Lupus 2015;24(2):180–5.

22. Ince-Askan H, Hazes JMW, Dolhain RJEM. Is disease activity in rheumatoid arthritis during pregnancy and after delivery predictive for disease activity in a subsequent pregnancy? J Rheumatol 2016;43:22–5.

23. Canti V, Castiglioni MT, Rosa S, et al. Pregnancy outcomes in patients with systemic autoimmunity. Autoimmunity 2012;45:169–75.

24. Clowse M, Magder LS, Witter F, et al. The impact of increased lupus activity on obstetric outcomes. Arthritis Rheum 2005;52(2):514–21.

25. Kwok LW, Tam LS, Zhu TY, et al. Predictors of maternal and fetal outcomes in pregnancies of patients with systemic lupus erythematosus. Lupus 2011;20:829–36.

26. Imbasciati E, Tincani A, Gregorini G, et al. Pregnancy in women with pre-existing lupus nephritis: predictors of fetal and maternal outcome. Nephrol Dial Transplant 2009;24:519–25.

27. Smyth A, Oliveira GH, Lahr BD, et al. A systematic review and meta-analysis of pregnancy outcomes in patients with systemic lupus erythematosus and lupus nephritis. Clin J Am Soc Nephrol 2010;5(11):2060–8.

28. Wallenius M, Salvesen KÅ, Daltveit AK, et al. Miscarriage and stillbirth in women with rheumatoid arthritis. J Rheumatol 2015;42:1570–2.

29. Brouwer J, Lavens JS, Hazes JM, et al. Miscarriages in females with rheumatoid arthritis patients:associations with serologic findings, disease activity and antirheumatic drug treatment. Arthritis Rheum 2015;67:1728–43.

30. Rom AL, Wu CS, Olsen J, et al. Fetal growth and preterm birth in children exposed to maternal or paternal rheumatoid arthritis: a nationwide cohort study. Arthritis Rheum 2014;68:3265–73.

31. de Man YA, Hazes JM, van der Helm H, et al. Association of higher rheumatoid arthritis disease activity during pregnancy with lower birth weight: results from a national prospective study. Arthritis Rheum 2009;60:3196–206.

32. Bowden AP, Barrett JH, Fallow W, et al. Women with inflammatory polyarthritis have babies of lower birth weight. J Rheumatol 2001;28:355–9.

33. Tingström J, Hjelmstedt A, Welin Henriksson E, et al. Anti-Ro/SSA autoantibody-positive women's experience of information given on the risk of congenital heart block. Lupus 2016;25(5):536–42.

34. Miyakis S, Lockshin MD, Atsumi T, et al. International consensus statement on an update of the classification criteria for definite antiphospholipid syndrome (APS). J Thromb Haemost 2006;4:295–306.

35. Nodler J, Moolamalla SR, Ledger EM, et al. Elevated antiphospholipid antibody titers and adverse pregnancy outcomes: analysis of a population-based hospital dataset. BMC Pregnancy Childbirth 2009;9:11–31.

36. Ruffatti A, Calligaro A, Hoxha A, et al. Laboratory and clinical features of pregnant women with antiphospholipid syndrome and neonatal outcome. Arthritis Care Res 2010;62:302–7.

37. Lockshin M, Kim M, Laskin CA, et al. Prediction of adverse pregnancy outcome by the presence of lupus anticoagulant, but not anticardiolipin antibody, in patients with antiphospholipid antibodies. Arthritis Rheum 2012;64:2311–8.

38. de Man YA, Bakker-Jonges LE, Goorbergh CM, et al. Women with rheumatoid arthritis negative for anti-cyclic citrullinated peptide and rheumatoid factor are more likely to improve during pregnancy, whereas in autoantibody-positive women autoantibody levels are not influenced by pregnancy. Ann Rheum Dis 2010;69:420–3.

39. Chakravarty E, Clowse MEB, Pushparajah DS, et al. Family planning and pregnancy issues for women with systemic inflammatory diseases: patient and physician perspectives. BMJ Open 2014;4:e004081.

40. Hämeen-Anttila K, Jyrkkä J, Enlund H, et al. Medicines information needs during pregnancy: a multinational comparison. BMJ Open 2013;3. http://dx.doi.org/10.1136/bmjopen-2013-002594.

41. Vinet E, Kuriya B, Pineau CA, et al. Induced abortions in women with rheumatoid arthritis receiving methotrexate. Arthritis Care Res 2013;65(8):1365–9.

42. Flint J, Panchal S, Hurrel M, et al. Audit Working, 2016, BSR and BHPR guideline on prescribing drugs in pregnancy and breastfeeding-Part I: standard and biologic disease modifying anti-rheumatic drugs and corticosteroids. Rheumatology (Oxford) 2016;55(9):1693–7.

43. Götestam Skorpen C, Hoeltzenbein M, Tincani A, et al. The EULAR points to consider for use of antirheumatic drugs before pregnancy, and during pregnancy and lactation. Ann Rheum Dis 2016;75:798–810.

44. Burdan F, Starosławska E, Szumiło J. Prenatal tolerability of acetaminophen and other over-the-counter non-selective cyclooxygenase inhibitors. Pharmacol Rep 2012;64(3):521–7.

45. Carlhäll S, Bladh M, Brynhildsen J, et al. Maternal obesity (Class I-III), gestational weight gain and maternal leptin levels during and after pregnancy: a prospective cohort study. BMC Obes 2016;3:28.
46. Czeizel AE, Dudás I, Vereczkey A, et al. Folate deficiency and folic acid supplementation: the prevention of neural-tube defects and congenital heart defects. Nutrients 2013;5(11):4760–75.

Biomarkers for Adverse Pregnancy Outcomes in Rheumatic Diseases

 CrossMark

May Ching Soh, FRACP[a,b,c,*],
Catherine Nelson-Piercy, FRCP, FRCOG[b,c]

KEYWORDS

- Adverse pregnancy outcomes • Preeclampsia • Growth restriction
- Soluble fms-like tyrosine kinase-1 • Placental growth factor • SLE
- Cardiovascular disease • Endothelial damage

KEY POINTS

- Adverse pregnancy outcomes are more common in women with rheumatic diseases, and the pathophysiology is likely multifactorial; hence, sole reliance on biomarkers to predict preterm delivery or other adverse outcomes may not be possible or advisable.
- Preterm (or classic) preeclampsia is a manifestation of placental insufficiency, which may also lead to fetal growth restriction, placental abruption, and stillbirth: collectively known as maternal-placental syndrome (MPS).
- Pregnancy is a delicate balance of circulating angiogenic factors of which antiangiogenic factors, for example, soluble fms-like tyrosine kinase-1 (sFlt-1) and soluble endoglin (sEng) predominate when there is MPS.
- Commercially available biomarkers, such as placental growth factor, sFlt-1, and sEng have the same diagnostic accuracy and prognostic significance in women with rheumatic diseases and chronic kidney disease as in healthy pregnant women.
- In the long term, the effect of these antiangiogenic biomarkers and the inflammatory cascade triggered by MPS, combined with preexisting metabolic risk factors, is likely contributory to the accelerated cardiovascular disease seen in young women with rheumatic diseases, especially systemic lupus erythematosus.

Dr M.C. Soh does not have any financial disclosures or conflicts of interest. Professor C. Nelson-Piercy has received speaker's fees and consultancy fees from UCB.
[a] Silver Star High-Risk Pregnancy Unit, John Radcliffe Hospital, Oxford University Hospitals NHS Foundation Trust, Headley Way, Oxford OX3 9DU, UK; [b] de Sweit Obstetric Medicine Department, Queen Charlotte's & Chelsea Hospital, Imperial College Healthcare NHS Trust, Du Cane Road, London W12 0HS, UK; [c] Women's Health Academic Centre, King's College London, St Thomas' Hospital, 10th Floor, North Wing, Westminster Bridge Road, London SE1 7EH, UK
* Corresponding author.
E-mail address: may_ching.soh@kcl.ac.uk

DEFINITIONS OF ADVERSE OUTCOMES IN PREGNANCY

Most autoimmune rheumatic diseases disproportionately affect women of child-bearing ages, and when pregnant, these women are at an increased risk of adverse pregnancy outcomes. Much of the published literature focuses on preeclampsia, a heterogeneous disorder identified by a common phenotype of hypertension and proteinuria. The crux of the disorder is the placenta, a highly vascular structure, and it is placental ischemia and insufficiency that gives rise to the recognized clinical manifestations. Therefore, future vascular disease is likely to initially manifest with clinical features of placental dysfunction or insufficiency. These features include the following:

i. Preeclampsia: new-onset hypertension and proteinuria in excess of 0.3 g/24 hours or $\geq$30 mg/mL on a spot urinary protein:creatinine urine sample after 20 weeks' gestation. It affects 3% to 5% of all pregnancies.[1]
ii. Fetal growth restriction: slowing or cessation of fetal growth while in utero.
iii. Small-for-gestational age (SGA) neonates: neonatal weight is lower than the 10th percentile of that expected for the population.
iv. Placental abruption: pathologic separation of the placenta from the uterus.
v. Stillbirth.

These features are often collectively known as maternal-placental syndrome (MPS). The individual features are not exclusive to MPS but also can occur for a variety of reasons, such as fetal chromosomal abnormalities or multiple pregnancies. Nevertheless, women with underlying rheumatic disease have a much higher incidence of these complications.[2]

Risk factors for preeclampsia and subsequent development of placental insufficiency are summarized in **Box 1**.

Box 1
Common risk factors for preeclampsia and subsequent placental insufficiency

- Nulliparity

- Extremes of maternal age younger than 18 years or older than 35 years

- Immunologic:
  - Multiparous women who have changed partner from previous pregnancies
  - Short interval between first coitus and conception
  - "Dangerous" father: man who has previously fathered preeclamptic pregnancies in a different woman.
  - Artificial reproductive therapy, especially with donor ovum

- Genetic: "familial clustering": inheritability of preeclampsia in twin studies is 22% to 47%

- Metabolic and vascular risk factors: for example, diabetes, obesity, chronic hypertension, renal dysfunction

- Thrombophilias, especially antiphospholipid syndrome

- Underlying autoimmune inflammatory diseases; for example, systemic lupus erythematosus, scleroderma

- Past factors:
  - Previous severe early-onset preeclampsia
  - Maternal preterm delivery
  - Maternal low birth weight

- Hypoxia:
  - Multifetal gestation
  - High altitude
  - Prolonged gestation: placental growth outstrips the vascular supply

---

In 2014, the International Society for the Study of Hypertension in Pregnancy revised the definition of preeclampsia to also include both maternal and fetal factors. The consequences of placental insufficiency can be best summarized in **Fig. 1**. The presence of proteinuria is not necessarily a diagnostic requirement if other systemic features of placental dysfunction (see **Fig. 1**) are present. There is evidence that women who develop nonproteinuric preeclampsia are more likely to have severe hypertension and exhibit other features of placental insufficiency leading to preterm deliveries.[3] Moreover, the severity of proteinuria has limited prognostic implications for pregnancy outcomes, and therefore quantification of proteinuria should not be repeated once the diagnosis of preeclampsia is established.[4]

PATHOPHYSIOLOGY OF PREECLAMPSIA

The classic hypothesis for preeclampsia is that it occurs as a result of defective placentation from ineffective spiral artery remodeling leading to placental hypoxia and the downstream cascade of all other clinical features, including fetal growth restriction with resultant infants who are SGA (see **Fig. 1**). Therefore, raised midgestational uterine artery Doppler studies are a useful marker for predicting preeclampsia-associated placental insufficiency. Nevertheless, the origins of classic preeclampsia are postulated to occur much earlier, even before conception, via paternal contribution (of semen or sperm) to impaired maternal immunotolerance.[5] Professor Redman subdivides the pathophysiological stages of classic or preterm preeclampsia into at least 6 steps[6,7] (**Table 1**). Women with rheumatic diseases are predisposed to poor placentation, and are therefore more likely to develop "classic" or preterm preeclampsia along with the vascular compromise and resultant fetal growth restriction.

However, the pathophysiological process of classic preterm preeclampsia does not explain the distinct clinical entity of "term preeclampsia," which is when preeclampsia occurs close to term or postterm. Fetal growth is usually unaffected in term preeclampsia, and therefore unlikely to be a result of defective placentation.[8]

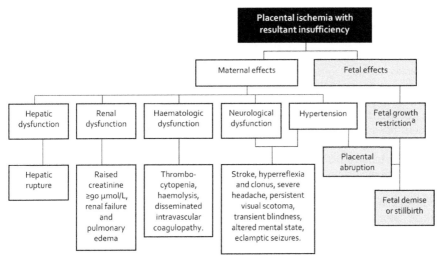

Fig. 1. Maternal and fetal consequences of placental dysfunction or MPS. [a] The effects of fetal growth restriction are more prominent in those who develop preeclampsia earlier in pregnancy. In term preeclampsia, the fetus has achieved its growth potential, therefore the effects of placental insufficiency from preeclampsia in fetal growth are less prominent.

Table 1
Six stages of "classic" preeclampsia

Stage 1	Before conception	Short interval between coitus to conception leads to lack of maternal immunotolerance to paternal antigens found in sperm or semen.
Stage 2 (<8 wk)	Implantation	Development of the embryo (little evidence of this at this stage).
Stage 3 (8–18 wk)	Defective placentation	Inadequate spiral artery remodeling and ischemic reperfusion and oxidative stress.
Stage 4 (>20 wk)	Oxidatively stressed placenta	Impaired production of placental-derived factors.
Stage 5	Overt clinical signs	Clinical manifestations of preeclampsia from placental insufficiency. The earlier the onset of stage 5, the more severe the fetal growth restriction.
Stage 6	Worsening preeclampsia with further compromise of uteroplacental perfusion	Acute atherosis (similar to atherosclerotic disease in later life) of the spiral arteries leading thrombosis and placental infarction/abruption.

Term preeclampsia starts at the later phases of stage 5 without antecedent defects in placentation. As it is of much later onset, fetal growth is unaffected, although the women will have other clinical features, such as hypertension or proteinuria. This is further exacerbated by falling placental growth factors and rising soluble fms-like tyrosine kinase-1 as the gestation advances.

The evidence lies in the normal midgestational (18–23^{+6} weeks) Doppler studies seen in this group who proceed to have normal-sized (if not large for gestational age) infants.[9,10] The underlying process is postulated to be physiologic in origin; in advanced gestation, the placenta "outgrows" its vascular supply, leading to a hypoxic environment that drives the pathophysiological processes of preeclampsia[8] (**Fig. 2**). This phenomenon is akin to a potted plant's roots outgrowing its pot (C.W. Redman, personal communication, 2016).

Maternal cardiovascular risk factors, for example, obesity, preexisting hypertension, dyslipidemia, metabolic syndrome, and other inflammatory diseases that accelerate vascular inflammation (ie, systemic lupus erythematosus [SLE] and other autoimmune connective tissue disorders) exacerbate the vascular inflammation at every stage and likely perpetuate the inflammation at stage 6, leading to accelerated cardiovascular events seen in women with placental dysfunction. A population-based study found that women who developed preeclampsia were more likely to have preexisting cardiovascular risk factors, such as hypertension and dyslipidemia. There was a correlation between the cardiovascular risk factors and severity of the preeclampsia.[11,12]

As hypertensive disorders in pregnancy also predispose a woman to developing future vascular disease, the American Heart Association now includes pregnancy complications in the form of hypertensive disorders of pregnancy, preeclampsia, and gestational diabetes mellitus as a major risk factor (within the same category of risk as having systemic autoimmune collagen vascular disease; eg, SLE and rheumatoid arthritis) for cardiovascular disease in women.[13]

Pregnancy itself is a low-grade, proinflammatory state that is exacerbated by the release of cellular syncytiotrophoblasts and other cellular debris from a damaged or ischemic placenta due to preeclampsia. These molecules can directly damage the endothelium or trigger a self-perpetuating maternal systemic inflammatory response cycle[14,15] (see **Fig. 2**). This cascade is driven by the complex interplay of placental

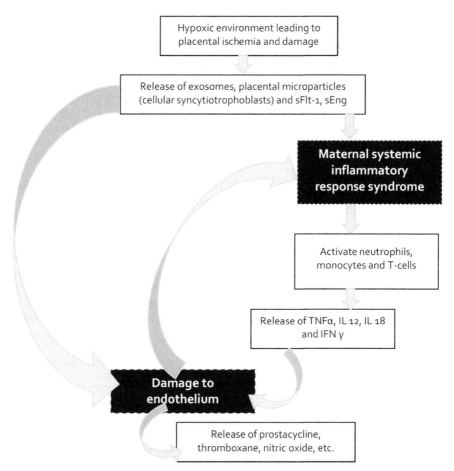

Fig. 2. Pathophysiology of preeclampsia. IFN, interferon; IL, interleukin.

angiogenic and antiangiogenic factors that are weighted in MPS in favor of an antiangiogenic state.

BIOMARKERS FOR THE PREDICTION OF PREECLAMPSIA

With the exception of low-dose aspirin (75–150 mg per day), which has only a moderate effect for the prevention of preeclampsia, there remains a lack of effective interventions for preventing and treating preeclampsia (or placental insufficiency) in women who are at high risk. There has been considerable effort invested in identifying biomarkers for the prediction of adverse pregnancy outcomes as a result of placental insufficiency. It is generally acknowledged that combinations of biomarkers perform better than single markers.[16,17]

Various studies have tried to combine a variety of factors, including past pregnancy outcomes, uterine or umbilical artery Doppler wave analysis, mean arterial pressure, maternal pregnancy-associated plasma protein A (PAPPA), placental protein 13 (PP 13), inhibin A, activin A, soluble endoglin (sEng), soluble fms-tyrosine kinase molecule-1 (sFlt-1), placental growth factor (PlGF), pentraxin-3, p-selectin, and many others in an attempt to predict and prognosticate placental insufficiency. Both sFlt-1 and PlGF are derived from syncytiotrophoblasts of the placenta.[18]

The focus of our review article is on the major biomarkers that have been shown to be of prognostic benefit and are currently commercially available.

PLACENTAL GROWTH FACTOR

Vascular endothelial growth factors (VEGFs) include PIGF and VEGF-A; both are released by the placenta. In the context of pregnancy and the placenta, VEGF has a direct vasodilatory effect (due to its effects on nitric oxide–dependent vessel relaxation). PIGF is expressed at high levels in the placenta, but also occurs in nonparous states. In pregnancy, PIGF levels increase from the second trimester and peak between 29 and 32 weeks.[19] In pregnancies complicated by preeclampsia, PIGF levels are low and correlate with severity of clinical presentation. It is likely that in the presence of hypoxia from placental insufficiency, the "stressed" syncytiotrophoblasts fail to produce adequate amounts of PIGF.

Using Triage PIGF (Alere International, Waltham, MA), which has a test limit of detection of 9 pg/mL, the recommended cutoff values are listed on **Table 2**.

Using PIGF with a less than fifth percentile for gestational age as a diagnostic cutoff for diagnosing preeclampsia, the PELICAN study, a prospective study performed in the United Kingdom and Ireland (n = 625), found that it had high sensitivity (0.96; 95% confidence interval [CI] 0.89–0.99) and negative predictive value (0.98; 95% CI 0.93–0.995) for preeclampsia within 14 days in women between 20 and 35 weeks' gestation.[20]

In the same PELICAN study, researchers found that a low serum PIGF (<12 pg/mL on Triage PIGF testing) was also useful for the prediction of preeclampsia necessitating preterm (<35 week) delivery within 14 days (adjusted hazard ratio controlling for gestational age and final diagnosis of 10.61; 95% CI 7.09–15.89).[21] This test was less useful when attempting to risk-stratify women after gestational age of 35 weeks for imminent delivery. PIGF levels vary according to gestational age and therefore a single cutoff is not available.

VEGF is also low in preeclampsia, but this is not a useful biomarker in clinical practice, as its levels are below detection in most of the currently available enzyme-linked immunosorbent assay kits.

SOLUBLE FMS-LIKE TYROSINE KINASE-1

sFlt-1, also known as soluble VEGF receptor-1 (sVEGFR-1), is an antiangiogenic factor that is a potent inhibitor of PIGF and VEGF. It is predominantly released by a hypoxic placenta (and its microparticles), but is also released by peripheral mononuclear cells, macrophages, and endothelial cells.

Table 2
Placental growth factor (PIGF) results and prognostic implications using Alere International's Triage PIGF test

PIGF Result, pg/mL	Classification	Prognostic Implications
<12	Highly abnormal	Severe placental dysfunction and at risk of preterm delivery
12–99	Abnormal	Suggestive of placental dysfunction and at risk of preterm delivery
≥100	Normal	Patients without placental dysfunction are unlikely to progress to preterm delivery within 14 d of the test

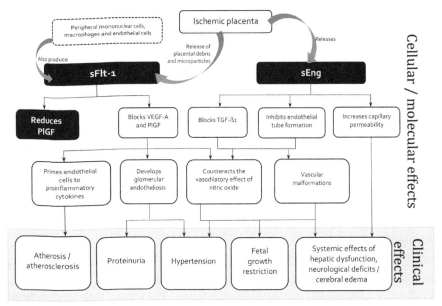

Fig. 4. Interaction of the 3 major biomarkers on the pathogenesis of MPS.

THE USE OF COMBINATION BIOMARKERS TO PREDICT ADVERSE OUTCOMES

Given the delicate balance of angiogenesis in pregnancy (see **Fig. 3**), biomarkers that work in combination may prove more useful than single markers for prediction of adverse pregnancy outcomes.[17] The combination biomarkers sFlt-1, sEng, and PlGF have an added value for the risk prediction for the need for preterm delivery in growth-restricted fetuses above that provided by clinical assessment and/or Doppler parameters.[25]

PROGNOSIS, a prospective international cohort study (n = 1500), has demonstrated that an sFlt-1/PlGF ratio less than 38 has an excellent negative predictive value in excluding preeclampsia in women between 24 and 36^{+6} weeks' gestation of 99.3% (95% CI 97.9–99.9), with 80.0% sensitivity (95% CI 51.9–95.7) and 78.3% specificity (95% CI 74.6–81.7).[26] Its negative predictive value was maximal in excluding

Table 3
Biomarkers in normal and preeclamptic pregnancies

Biomarker	Normal Pregnancy[a]	Pregnancy Affected by "Classic" or Preterm Preeclampsia
PlGF	Increase from second trimester and peak at 29–32 wk, then decline.	Low levels
sFlt-1	Remains constant until approximately 30–32 wk, then gradually rises toward term.	Increase in levels 5 wk before onset of clinical symptoms of preeclampsia.
sEng	Starts to increase from 33 wk until delivery.	Increasing levels from 20 wk of gestation (in preterm preeclampsia).

Abbreviations: PlGF, placental growth factor; sEng, soluble endoglin; sFlt-1, soluble fms-like tyrosine kinase-1.
[a] In term preeclampsia, the biomarkers follow the similar profile of a normal pregnancy.

In normal pregnancy, sFlt-1 is present at high concentrations at term and de
48 hours after delivery of the placenta. However, it is also detectable 5 v
before the onset of clinical preeclampsia and correlates with the severi
preeclampsia.

sFLt-1 exerts its effects in several ways (**Fig. 3**). First, it blocks VEGF and F
therefore inhibiting vasodilation with a resultant increase in maternal systemic vaso
resistance or blood pressure. It also primes endothelial cells to proinflammatory c
kines, such as tumor necrosis factor (TNF). Finally, it contributes to the developmen
proteinuria seen in preeclampsia by promoting the development of glomerular ca
lary endotheliosis, a histopathologic finding on renal biopsies seen in kidneys
women with preeclampsia (**Fig. 4**).

Although sFlt-1 raises the maternal blood pressure and promotes proteinuria
does not have any effect on the more systemic features of preeclampsia, such as
patic and neurologic dysfunction or fetal growth restriction.

SOLUBLE ENDOGLIN

sEng is a cell-surface coreceptor of transforming growth factor-β1 (TGF-β
and TGF-β3. In the nonparous state, sEng is associated with endothelial dysfunc
tion and dyslipidemia and cardiovascular events.[22] In normal pregnancies, level
are stable until approximately 33 weeks when levels increase and peak at delivery
In preterm preeclampsia, levels of sEng start increasing from approximately
20 weeks' gestation, and it is present in much higher levels than a normal pregnancy (**Table 3**).

sEng blocks TGF-β1–mediated vasodilation, inhibits endothelial tube formation with
resultant vascular malformations, and increases capillary permeability (see **Fig. 3**).
Raised sEng levels correlate with increased impedance of flow to uterine and umbilical
artery Dopplers.[23] In mouse models, sEng is also associated with decreased cerebral
perfusion and edema. Therefore, it is associated with the more severe features of preeclampsia and fetal growth restriction.

sEng is closely correlated with sFlt-1 and PlGF levels in women with preeclampsia,
and its presence is associated with a 10-fold increased risk of fetal growth
restriction.[24]

These biomarkers and their levels in both normal and preeclamptic pregnancies are
summarized in **Table 3**.

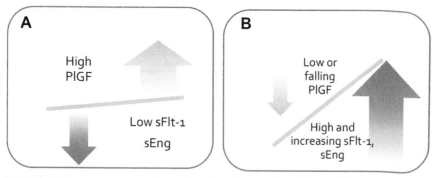

Fig. 3. The balance of common biomarkers for placental insufficiency (*A*) In a normal pregnancy (or <30 wk gestation), (*B*) In a pre-eclamptic pregnancy (or as the pregnancy pro-
gresses toward term).

preeclampsia within 7 days of the test, but performed less well, with sensitivity of only 66.2% (95% CI 54.0–77.0), to rule-in preeclampsia within 4 weeks of the test.

In the United Kingdom, the National Institute for Health and Care Excellence (NICE) recently published diagnostic guidance on the use of angiogenic markers to aid in the diagnosis of preeclampsia[27] (https://www.nice.org.uk/guidance/dg23). Although NICE suggested that the Triage PIGF test and the Elecsys immunoassay sFlt-1/PIGF ratio, when used with standard clinical assessment and clinical follow-up, show promise in helping to diagnose (rule-in) preeclampsia in those presenting with suspected preeclampsia between 20^{+0} and 34^{+6} weeks' gestation, there remains insufficient evidence to recommend their routine adoption in clinical practice.

UTILITY OF BIOMARKERS IN PREEXISTING HYPERTENSION AND CHRONIC KIDNEY DISEASE

The diagnosis of preeclampsia in women with preexisting hypertension and chronic kidney disease (CKD) is fraught with difficulties, as both elevated blood pressure and proteinuria, the most common clinical features of preeclampsia, are already present in this high-risk cohort of women. Moreover, proteinuria tends to gradually worsen with advancing gestation and it is difficult to differentiate preeclampsia from the increasing physiologic demands of pregnancy on the kidney.

Bramham and colleagues[28] validated the use of these biomarkers in these high-risk women (n = 161 women with CKD and chronic hypertension) in a longitudinal cohort study. The researchers found that both sFlt-1 and PIGF could be used in a similar fashion as the normal population (ie, without preexisting maternal hypertension or CKD). In particular, a low PIGF had a high diagnostic accuracy for predicting delivery within 14 days of the test for superimposed preeclampsia. The addition of sFlt-1 (or an sFlt-1/PIGF ratio >85) did not provide incremental value for the prediction of preeclampsia over and above a low PIGF (<5th percentile) alone.

UTILITY OF BIOMARKERS IN RHEUMATIC DISEASES, PARTICULARLY SYSTEMIC LUPUS ERYTHEMATOSUS

SLE is the commonest autoimmune disease affecting women of childbearing age. Therefore, most studies on biomarkers for adverse pregnancy outcomes in women with rheumatic disease have involved women with SLE.

An early nested case-control study by Dr Petri's group demonstrated that sFlt-1 is increased in patients with SLE with preeclampsia.[29] All other biomarkers (sFlt-1, PIGF, and sEng) were useful in predicting early-onset preeclampsia in women with SLE when measured at 12 weeks of gestation.[30] These early findings were validated by the PROMISSE study, a large international cohort study, which confirmed that sFlt-1 measured between 12 and 15 weeks of gestation was the strongest predictor of adverse pregnancy outcomes in women with SLE and/or antiphospholipid syndrome, whereas sFlt and PIGF were more useful for prognosticating pregnancy outcomes in those between 16 and 19 weeks of gestation.[31]

CLINICAL UTILITY IN RISK PREDICTION OF PREECLAMPSIA OR ADVERSE PREGNANCY OUTCOMES

Although the efficacy of aspirin in the prevention of preeclampsia and other features of MPS remains limited, the use of biomarkers to predict adverse pregnancy outcomes remains clinically relevant for the allocation of resources for intense antenatal surveillance necessary in women who are deemed to be at high risk. It is reassuring that these biomarkers perform with similar accuracy even in those with underlying maternal disease and in particular CKD and SLE.

Women who are at high risk of adverse pregnancy outcomes will require frequent review during pregnancy with regular growth scans and Doppler scans of their uterine/umbilical arteries to allow the timely diagnosis of MPS and optimize the timing of delivery in this group. This intensive antenatal surveillance is not just a matter of resource allocation in a financially restricted health care environment, but intensive follow-up also places a significant emotional burden on the woman. Hence, having biomarkers that can risk-stratify women according to likely outcomes early (<20 weeks gestation) means that clinicians are able to "normalize" the antenatal care for many lower risk women.

ARE ANGIOGENIC BIOMARKERS THE ANSWER FOR PREDICTION OF ADVERSE PREGNANCY OUTCOMES IN WOMEN WITH RHEUMATIC DISEASES?

Women with autoimmune rheumatic diseases have a heighted risk of adverse pregnancy outcomes compared with the normal population. Although angiogenic biomarkers play a significant role, it is likely that other factors, such as disease activity in pregnancy (and in the 4–6 months preceding pregnancy), preexisting end-organ damage, or medications used, also should be included in this risk stratification for adverse pregnancy outcomes. Moreover, women with rheumatic diseases are generally older, have more medical comorbidities, and are more likely to use artificial reproductive therapy when they do become pregnant. Hence, prediction of adverse pregnancy outcomes in these women cannot be based solely on biomarkers as in the general population.

ADVERSE PREGNANCY OUTCOMES AND FUTURE VASCULAR DISEASE

Appreciation of the role played by the placenta in future health, both for the mother and the fetus, is increasing.[32] Several chronic illnesses, particularly those associated with the metabolic syndrome and cardiovascular disease, have been linked to placental dysfunction.[33]

A meta-analysis of more than 3 million pregnancies has shown that preeclampsia is linked to an almost fourfold increased risk of subsequent hypertension, and a twofold increased risk of stroke and ischemic heart disease.[34] Other features of MPS, such as SGA, are associated with a 1.4-fold increased risk of cardiovascular events, a risk that increases as the duration of gestation decreases.[35] A Canadian population-based study (Cardiovascular Health After Maternal-Placental Syndrome study) demonstrated that the risk of cardiovascular disease was highest among those who had intrauterine death (hazard ratio 4.4, 95% CI 2.4–7.9).[36]

There are 2 hypotheses linking MPS and future cardiovascular events. First, preexisting vascular dysfunction may predispose the woman to abnormal placentation during pregnancy and this represents the link between placental insufficiency and the development of vascular disease later in life.[37,38] Women with preexisting cardiovascular risk factors, such as dyslipidemia and hypertension, are more likely to develop preeclampsia.[11] These women also tend to have shorter gestations.[39]

Alternatively, the endothelial damage from circulating angiogenic factors and other inflammatory molecules (see **Fig. 2**) after a pregnancy complicated by preeclampsia may be a predisposing factor for future vascular disease. Moreover, during delivery, separation of the placenta results in further shedding of cellular debris into the maternal circulation.[40] This cellular debris not only worsens preeclampsia in the immediate postpartum interval, but could further damage the systemic maternal endothelium.

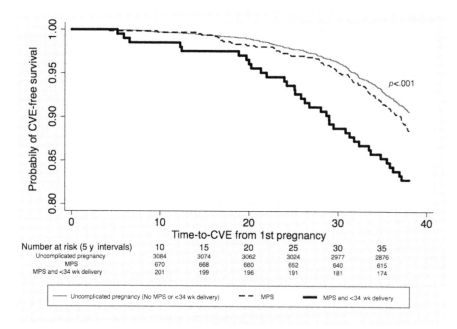

Fig. 5. Probability of cardiovascular event (CVE)-free survival after MPS in parous women with SLE. (*Reproduced from* Soh MC, Dib F, Nelson-Piercy C, et al. Maternal-placental syndrome and future risk of accelerated cardiovascular events in parous Swedish women with systemic lupus erythematosus—a population-based retrospective cohort study with time-to-event analysis. Rheumatology (Oxford) 2016;55(7):1240; with permission.)

Women with SLE have a much higher risk of premature cardiovascular disease and death compared with the normal population, even in the relative absence of any traditional cardiovascular risk factors.[41] Women who have had pregnancies complicated by MPS are at greater risk of death from cardiovascular causes and accelerated development of cardiovascular disease (**Fig. 5**).[2,42] Preterm delivery of fewer than 34 weeks, which could be a surrogate marker for active SLE in pregnancy, also has been associated with accelerated cardiovascular events in this cohort (data presented at 9th International Conference for Reproduction, Pregnancy and Rheumatic Diseases, San Diego, April 2016; http://www.rheumpreg2016.org/agenda.html).

Hence, pregnancy is a "stress test" for life. Clinicians caring for women with rheumatic diseases should include history of adverse pregnancy outcomes, especially MPS, when screening for cardiovascular risk factors. Actively managing other modifiable cardiovascular risk factors (eg, obesity, smoking, hypertension, and dyslipidemia) is especially important if the woman has had a past pregnancy complicated by MPS or a preterm delivery.

Further research on the role of angiogenic biomarkers in pregnancies and subsequent health in women with rheumatic diseases and the potential influence of biological therapies on these biomarkers is needed.

ACKNOWLEDGMENTS

The authors thank Professor Christopher W. Redman of John Radcliffe Hospital, Oxford University, for his amazing insight into the pathophysiology of preeclampsia, both classic and term preeclampsia.

REFERENCES

1. Chaiworapongsa T, Chaemsaithong P, Yeo L, et al. Pre-eclampsia part 1: current understanding of its pathophysiology. Nat Rev Nephrol 2014;10(8):466–80.
2. Soh MC, Nelson-Piercy C, Dib F, et al. Association between pregnancy outcomes and cardiovascular deaths in women with systemic lupus erythematosus utilising Swedish population registries. Arthritis Rheumatol (Hoboken, NJ) 2015;67(9): 2376–82.
3. Homer CS, Brown MA, Mangos G, et al. Non-proteinuric pre-eclampsia: a novel risk indicator in women with gestational hypertension. J Hypertens 2008;26(2): 295–302.
4. Thangaratinam S, Coomarasamy A, O'Mahony F, et al. Estimation of proteinuria as a predictor of complications of pre-eclampsia: a systematic review. BMC Med 2009;7:10.
5. Redman CW, Sargent IL. Immunology of pre-eclampsia. Am J Reprod Immunol 2010;63(6):534–43.
6. Redman CW. Pre-eclampsia: definitions, paternal contributions and a four stage model. Pregnancy Hypertens 2011;1(1):2–5.
7. Redman C. The six stages of pre-eclampsia. Pregnancy Hypertens 2014;4(3): 246.
8. Redman CW, Sargent IL, Staff AC. IFPA Senior Award Lecture: making sense of pre-eclampsia - two placental causes of preeclampsia? Placenta 2014; 35(Suppl):S20–5.
9. Verlohren S, Melchiorre K, Khalil A, et al. Uterine artery Doppler, birth weight and timing of onset of pre-eclampsia: providing insights into the dual etiology of late-onset pre-eclampsia. Ultrasound Obstet Gynecol 2014;44(3):293–8.
10. Rasmussen S, Irgens LM, Espinoza J. Maternal obesity and excess of fetal growth in pre-eclampsia. BJOG 2014;121(11):1351–7.
11. Magnussen EB, Vatten LJ, Lund-Nilsen TI, et al. Prepregnancy cardiovascular risk factors as predictors of pre-eclampsia: population based cohort study. BMJ 2007;335(7627):978.
12. Romundstad PR, Magnussen EB, Smith GD, et al. Hypertension in pregnancy and later cardiovascular risk: common antecedents? Circulation 2010;122(6): 579–84.
13. Mosca L, Benjamin EJ, Berra K, et al. Effectiveness-based guidelines for the prevention of cardiovascular disease in women–2011 update: a guideline from the American Heart Association. J Am Coll Cardiol 2011;57(12):1404–23.
14. Clifton VL, Stark MJ, Osei-Kumah A, et al. The feto-placental unit, pregnancy pathology and impact on long term maternal health. Placenta 2012;33(26):S37–41.
15. Redman CW, Sargent IL. Circulating microparticles in normal pregnancy and pre-eclampsia. Placenta 2008;29(Suppl A):S73–7.
16. Kuc S, Wortelboer EJ, van Rijn BB, et al. Evaluation of 7 serum biomarkers and uterine artery Doppler ultrasound for first-trimester prediction of preeclampsia: a systematic review. Obstet Gynecol Surv 2011;66(4):225–39.
17. Chaiworapongsa T, Chaemsaithong P, Korzeniewski SJ, et al. Pre-eclampsia part 2: prediction, prevention and management. Nat Rev Nephrol 2014;10(9):531–40.
18. Redman CW, Staff AC. Preeclampsia, biomarkers, syncytiotrophoblast stress, and placental capacity. Am J Obstet Gynecol 2015;213(4 Suppl):S9.e1. S9–S11.
19. Powe CE, Levine RJ, Karumanchi SA. Preeclampsia, a disease of the maternal endothelium: the role of antiangiogenic factors and implications for later cardiovascular disease. Circulation 2011;123(24):2856–69.

20. Chappell LC, Duckworth S, Seed PT, et al. Diagnostic accuracy of placental growth factor in women with suspected preeclampsia: a prospective multicenter study. Circulation 2013;128(19):2121–31.

21. Duckworth S, Chappell LC, Griffin M, et al. Plasma Placental Growth Factor (PlGF) in the diagnosis of women with pre-eclampsia requiring delivery within 14 days. BJOG 2013;120(9):E1–2.

22. Rathouska J, Jezkova K, Nemeckova I, et al. Soluble endoglin, hypercholesterolemia and endothelial dysfunction. Atherosclerosis 2015;243(2):383–8.

23. Chaiworapongsa T, Romero R, Kusanovic JP, et al. Plasma soluble endoglin concentration in pre-eclampsia is associated with an increased impedance to flow in the maternal and fetal circulations. Ultrasound Obstet Gynecol 2010;35(2):155–62.

24. Rana S, Cerdeira AS, Wenger J, et al. Plasma concentrations of soluble endoglin versus standard evaluation in patients with suspected preeclampsia. PLoS One 2012;7(10):e48259.

25. Chaiworapongsa T, Romero R, Whitten AE, et al. The use of angiogenic biomarkers in maternal blood to identify which SGA fetuses will require a preterm delivery and mothers who will develop pre-eclampsia. J Maternal Fetal Neonatal Med 2015;29(8):1214–28.

26. Zeisler H, Llurba E, Chantraine F, et al. Predictive value of the sFlt-1:PlGF ratio in women with suspected preeclampsia. N Engl J Med 2016;374(1):13–22.

27. The National Institute for Health and Care Excellence (NICE). PlGF-based testing to help diagnose suspected pre-eclampsia. (Diagnostic Guidance) 2016.

28. Bramham K, Seed PT, Lightstone L, et al. Diagnostic and predictive biomarkers for pre-eclampsia in patients with established hypertension and chronic kidney disease. Kidney Int 2016;89(4):874–85.

29. Qazi U, Lam C, Karumanchi SA, et al. Soluble fms-like tyrosine kinase associated with preeclampsia in pregnancy in systemic lupus erythematosus. J Rheumatol 2008;35(4):631–4.

30. Leanos-Miranda A, Campos-Galicia I, Berumen-Lechuga MG, et al. Circulating angiogenic factors and the risk of preeclampsia in systemic lupus erythematosus pregnancies. J Rheumatol 2015;42(7):1141–9.

31. Kim MY, Buyon JP, Guerra MM, et al. Angiogenic factor imbalance early in pregnancy predicts adverse outcomes in patients with lupus and antiphospholipid antibodies: results of the PROMISSE study. Am J Obstet Gynecol 2016;214(1):108.e1-e14.

32. Nelson DM. How the placenta affects your life, from womb to tomb. Am J Obstet Gynecol 2015;213(4 Suppl):S12–3.

33. Thornburg KL, Marshall N. The placenta is the center of the chronic disease universe. Am J Obstet Gynecol 2015;213(4 Suppl):S14–20.

34. Bellamy L, Casas JP, Hingorani AD, et al. Pre-eclampsia and risk of cardiovascular disease and cancer in later life: systematic review and meta-analysis. BMJ 2007;335(7627):974.

35. Bonamy AK, Parikh NI, Cnattingius S, et al. Birth characteristics and subsequent risks of maternal cardiovascular disease: effects of gestational age and fetal growth. Circulation 2011;124(25):2839–46.

36. Ray JG, Vermeulen MJ, Schull MJ, et al. Cardiovascular health after maternal placental syndromes (CHAMPS): population-based retrospective cohort study. Lancet 2005;366(9499):1797–803.

37. Roberts JM, Redman CW. Pre-eclampsia: more than pregnancy-induced hypertension. Lancet 1993;341(8858):1447–51.

38. Roberts JM, Cooper DW. Pathogenesis and genetics of pre-eclampsia. Lancet 2001;357(9249):53–6.
39. Magnussen EB, Vatten LJ, Myklestad K, et al. Cardiovascular risk factors prior to conception and the length of pregnancy: population-based cohort study. Am J Obstet Gynecol 2011;204(6):526.e1-e8.
40. Reddy A, Zhong XY, Rusterholz C, et al. The effect of labour and placental separation on the shedding of syncytiotrophoblast microparticles, cell-free DNA and mRNA in normal pregnancy and pre-eclampsia. Placenta 2008;29(11):942–9.
41. Urowitz MB, Gladman D, Ibanez D, et al. Atherosclerotic vascular events in a multinational inception cohort of systemic lupus erythematosus. Arthritis Care Res (Hoboken) 2010;62(6):881–7.
42. Soh MC, Dib F, Nelson-Piercy C, et al. Maternal-placental syndrome and future risk of accelerated cardiovascular events in parous Swedish women with systemic lupus erythematosus—a population-based retrospective cohort study with time-to-event analysis. Rheumatology (Oxford) 2016;55(7):1235–42.

Systemic Lupus Erythematosus and Pregnancy

Aisha Lateef, MBBS, MRCP, MMed, FAMS[a], Michelle Petri, MD, MPH[b],*

KEYWORDS

- Systemic lupus erythematosus • Antibodies • Pregnancy • Fetal loss
- Preeclampsia • Neonatal lupus syndromes

KEY POINTS

- Outcomes for pregnancy in the setting of systemic lupus erythematosus have considerably improved but the maternal and fetal risks still remain high.
- Disease flares, preeclampsia, pregnancy loss, preterm births, intrauterine growth restriction, and neonatal lupus syndromes (especially heart block) remain the main complications.
- Specific monitoring and treatment protocols need to be used for situations such as presence of specific antibodies (antiphospholipid antibodies and anti-Ro/La).
- Safe and effective treatment options exist and should be used as appropriate to control disease activity during pregnancy.
- Close monitoring, tailored multidisciplinary care, and judicious use of medications are the key to achieve optimal outcomes.

INTRODUCTION

Systemic lupus erythematosus (SLE) is a multisystem autoimmune disease with a strong female predilection. Disease onset in a younger age group, coupled with improved survival, makes pregnancy a likely occurrence in the setting of SLE. Although outcomes have improved over time and successful live births can now be achieved in most cases, pregnancy still remains a high-risk situation in SLE.[1–3] Both maternal and fetal mortality and morbidity are significantly increased, along with health care utilization and costs.[2–5] A multidisciplinary coordinated approach with

Disclosures: The authors have no commercial or financial conflict of interest and no funding source for this work.
[a] Division of Rheumatology, University Medicine Cluster, National University Hospital, National University Health System, 1E, Kent Ridge Road, Singapore 119074; [b] Division of Rheumatology, Johns Hopkins Lupus Center, Johns Hopkins University School of Medicine, 1830 East Monument Street, Suite 7500, Baltimore, MD 21205, USA
* Corresponding author.
E-mail address: mpetri@jhmi.edu

Rheum Dis Clin N Am 43 (2017) 215–226
http://dx.doi.org/10.1016/j.rdc.2016.12.009
0889-857X/17/© 2017 Elsevier Inc. All rights reserved.

rheumatic.theclinics.com

involvement of appropriate specialists and close monitoring is essential for optimal outcomes. This article discusses major issues and the management principles to guide clinicians caring for pregnant women with SLE.

EFFECTS OF PREGNANCY ON SYSTEMIC LUPUS ERYTHEMATOSUS DISEASE ACTIVITY

Although opinions differ, most studies have shown that risk of SLE flare is higher during pregnancy. Variable flare rates of between 25% to 65% have been reported, likely attributable to different study designs, patient populations, and assessment tools being used.[6–8] Multiple predictors for flares have been identified, including disease activity at the time of conception, lupus nephritis, and discontinuation of medications such as hydroxychloroquine (HCQ).[9,10] Most of these flares are mild to moderate in severity and involve renal, musculoskeletal, and hematological systems.[11] Recognition and management of the flares during pregnancy can be challenging because features may be altered and therapeutic options limited.

Recognition of Disease Activity During Pregnancy

Recognition of disease activity and flare in pregnancy can be difficult because physiologic changes of pregnancy may overlap with features of active disease (**Table 1**). Investigations have to be interpreted with caution: mild degrees of anemia, thrombocytopenia, proteinuria, and increased erythrocyte sedimentation rate are common during pregnancy. Complement levels become less informative with the increase in levels during normal pregnancy. The trend becomes more important, and decline in levels of complement during pregnancy has been associated with poor pregnancy outcomes.[12,13] The use of SLE disease activity indices faces similar issues, because physiologic pregnancy changes were not accounted for in these tools. Pregnancy-specific disease activity scales have been developed but utility remains limited. The clinical judgment of an experienced physician may the best tool to evaluate disease activity in some scenarios.

Management of Disease Activity Pregnancy

Treatment of disease activity and flares during pregnancy requires the use of medications that are effective but safe for the growing fetus. However, patients and sometimes even physicians discontinue medications because of concerns over

Table 1
Overlapping features of pregnancy and systemic lupus erythematosus

	Pregnancy Changes	SLE Activity
Clinical Features	Facial flush	Photosensitive rash
	Palmar erythema	Oral or nasal ulcers
	Arthralgias	Inflammatory arthritis
	Fatigue	Fatigue, lethargy
	Mild edema	Moderate to severe edema
	Mild resting dyspnea	Pleuritis
Laboratory Features	Mild anemia	Immune hemolytic anemia
	Mild thrombocytopenia	Thrombocytopenia
		Leukopenia, lymphopenia
	Mildly increased ESR	Increased inflammatory marker levels
	Physiologic proteinuria <300 mg/d	Proteinuria >300 mg/d
		Active urinary sediment

Abbreviation: ESR, erythrocyte sedimentation rate.

presumed toxicity, resulting in avoidable disease flares and associated consequences. The fear is compounded by lack of information because the data on safety of drugs during pregnancy are generally limited to registries, case reports, or animal studies. However, although choices are limited and maternal benefit has to be weighed against fetal toxicity, multiple effective options exist and should be used[14,15] (**Table 2**).

Steroids can be continued during pregnancy for optimal disease control but attempts should be made to minimize the exposure. High doses of steroids are associated with an increased risk of diabetes, hypertension, preeclampsia, and premature rupture of membranes, but short-term use for flares and disease control is permissible.[14] Similarly, use of fluorinated compounds, such as dexamethasone and betamethasone, should be limited to single courses for fetal lung maturity in cases of premature delivery. Repeated use should be avoided in view of association with impaired neuropsychological development of the offspring in later life.[16]

HCQ has multiple proven benefits in SLE and continued use throughout pregnancy is strongly recommended. Pregnancy-specific benefits include reduction in disease activity, lower risk of flares, and reduced risk of heart block in at-risk pregnancies.[17–20] HCQ discontinuation was shown to increase disease flares during pregnancy and should be discouraged.[17]

Commonly used immunosuppressive agents, such as cyclophosphamide, methotrexate, and mycophenolate, have teratogenic potential and ideally should be discontinued before conception. Safe immunosuppressants for pregnancy use include azathioprine and the calcineurin inhibitors, tacrolimus and cyclosporine.[14,15] Multiple studies have shown them to be safe and effective therapies for use during pregnancy. An association between maternal azathioprine therapy and late developmental delays (specifically, increased use of special education services) in offspring was suggested by 1 study but remains to be confirmed.[21] Some risk of fetal cytopenias and immune suppression has been reported with higher doses and it is recommended to limit the dose to a maximum of 2 mg/kg/d.[14] Although safety of inadvertent exposure to leflunomide (usually followed by cholestyramine washout) has been reported, data are limited.[22,23] It should be discontinued before pregnancy with consideration of washout procedure.[15] Use of biologic drugs during pregnancy is increasing but is still limited to anti–tumor necrosis factor agents, which are not an option for SLE.[15,24] Data on other

Table 2 Immunosuppressant use during systemic lupus erythematosus pregnancy	
Drugs	**Comments**
Corticosteroids	Use lowest possible dose
• Prednisolone/pulse methyl prednisolone	Higher doses can lead to maternal complications
	Pulse therapy can be used for acute flares
• Fluorinated compounds (betamethasone/ dexamethasone)	Limit to 1 course, for fetal lung maturation
	Repeated use associated with impaired neuropsychological development of the child
Antimalarials	Reduced risk of disease flares, CHB, and NLS
• Hydroxychloroquine	Should be continued in all SLE pregnancies
Immunosuppressants	Limit azathioprine dose to 2 mg/kg/d
• Azathioprine	
• Calcineurin inhibitors (cyclosporine/tacrolimus)	

Abbreviations: CHB, complete heart block; NLS, neonatal lupus syndromes.

biologic agents, such as rituximab and belimumab, are very limited, and use should be limited to situations in which no other pregnancy-safe option is viable.[15] Intravenous immunoglobulin (IVIG) and plasmapheresis remain alternative options in selected situations.[15,25]

EFFECT OF SYSTEMIC LUPUS ERYTHEMATOSUS ON PREGNANCY OUTCOMES

The interaction of SLE, an immune-mediated disease, and immunologic adaptations of pregnancy lead to unique challenges in this setting. Both mother and baby are at high risk of adverse pregnancy outcomes (APOs), including preeclampsia, preterm delivery, pregnancy loss, and intrauterine growth restriction (IUGR). The predictors of APO include active maternal disease, nephritis, proteinuria, hypertension, thrombocytopenia, and presence of antiphospholipid antibodies (aPLs), especially lupus anticoagulant.[10,26–30] Ethnic differences have also been reported, likely reflective of racial differences in disease and access to health care.[10,31]

Pregnancy loss has declined significantly over the decades and live birth rates of 80% to 90% have been reported.[1,25] Preterm births are now the most frequent problem, occurring in up to half of the pregnancies with poor prognostic markers listed earlier. In addition, thyroid disease is associated with preterm birth in SLE pregnancy.[32]

Higher rates of maternal death, thrombosis, infection, and hematologic complications during SLE pregnancy have been reported, although nonpregnant patients with SLE also have higher risks of these medical complications and mortality.[2,3] Neurodevelopmental disorders in offspring of mothers with SLE represent an emerging concern that requires further study.[33,34]

Preeclampsia in Systemic Lupus Erythematosus Pregnancy

Preeclampsia affects 16% to 30% of SLE pregnancies compared with 5% to 7% in healthy women. In addition to the general predisposing factors (advanced maternal age, previous personal or family history of preeclampsia, preexisting hypertension or diabetes mellitus, obesity), SLE-specific predictors for preeclampsia include active or history of lupus nephritis, presence of aPLs, thrombocytopenia, declining complement levels, and mutations in complement regulatory proteins.[35–37]

The high risk of preeclampsia in SLE pregnancy is compounded by the difficulty in differentiating it from lupus nephritis. Both conditions can manifest with increasing proteinuria, deteriorating renal function, hypertension, and thrombocytopenia, and can even coexist. Guidelines and biomarkers have been proposed but have limited utility. Ultrasonography findings such as abnormal uterine artery waveforms have shown good utility as diagnostic tools, and predictive modeling has been attempted for early recognition.[38–40] However, all these measures have limitations and differentiation may be extremely difficult. Renal biopsy could guide management in selected cases and is safe in experienced hands.[41] However, at times, delivery of the baby may be the only definitive answer.

MANAGEMENT GUIDELINES FOR PREGNANCY IN SYSTEMIC LUPUS ERYTHEMATOSUS

Ideally, pregnancy should be timed during a period of disease quiescence because active disease at the time of conception is known to be one of the strongest predictors of APO. However, unplanned pregnancies are common, highlighting the often neglected need for contraceptive counseling in this group of women.[42] Effective contraceptive choices include combined oral contraceptives in women with stable disease and negative aPL, progesterone-only contraceptives, and intrauterine devices, whereas barrier methods are ineffective, with high failure rate (see Lisa R. Sammaritano's article, "Contraception in Rheumatic Disease Patients," in this issue).[43] Caution is required when making decisions regarding contraception in women with aPL and active disease in view of limited data.

Pregnancy may carry a very high maternal risk in a subset of patients with SLE, and should be avoided in these women (**Box 1**). However, successful pregnancy is possible for most women with SLE, albeit with a higher risk. Prepregnancy evaluation with assessment of autoantibody profile, end-organ function, disease activity, and medication use helps to risk stratify, identify optimal timing, and plan the management strategy for each pregnancy (**Fig. 1**).

All pregnant women with SLE should be closely monitored during pregnancy, preferably by a multidisciplinary team of appropriate specialists. A recent large study showed reduction in immunosuppression use and rheumatologist visits despite overall increased health care use during SLE pregnancies.[4] This finding again emphasizes the need for a team-based approach in the care of these high-risk pregnancies. Antenatal monitoring should be tailored to the individual needs of the patient but generally requires frequent review, especially in the presence of poor prognostic markers. Presence of certain antibodies poses special risk and deserves closer attention.

Antiphospholipid Antibodies in Systemic Lupus Erythematosus Pregnancy

aPLs are present in a quarter to half of patients with SLE. Some of these patients are asymptomatic, whereas others develop thrombotic or obstetric complications, termed the antiphospholipid syndrome (APS). The presence of aPL significantly increases the risk of APO, even in asymptomatic women.

Management of exposed pregnancies depends on the risk profile and can be categorized into 3 main groups. Asymptomatic carriers are women with positive aPL but no prior clinical event. Low-dose aspirin has been recommended but multiple studies have failed to show the benefit of this approach.[44–46] However, use of prophylactic aspirin in this setting remains common. The second group includes women with recurrent pregnancy losses but no systemic thrombosis, termed obstetric APS. Combination therapy with aspirin and prophylactic doses of heparin significantly reduces the risk of pregnancy loss in this group.[46,47] The third group is composed of patients with APS and prior systemic thrombosis. These women should receive full therapeutic doses of heparin throughout pregnancy. Heparin should be continued for 6 weeks postpartum. Low-molecular-weight heparin (LMWH) can be used in place of

---

Box 1
High maternal risk situations for pregnancy in systemic lupus erythematosus

Avoid pregnancy if:

Severe pulmonary hypertension (systolic pulmonary artery pressure >50 mm Hg)

Severe restrictive lung disease (forced vital capacity <1 L)

Advanced renal insufficiency (creatinine level >2.8 mg/dL)

Advance heart failure

Previous severe preeclampsia or HELLP (hemolysis, elevated liver enzyme levels, low platelet count) despite therapy

Stroke within the previous 6 months

Severe disease flare within last 6 months

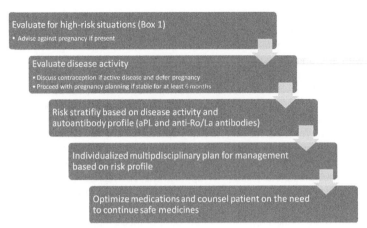

Fig. 1. Prepregnancy evaluation for patients with SLE.

unfractionated heparin because it has comparable efficacy but fewer adverse effects with easier monitoring.

The outcomes of aPL-exposed pregnancies have significantly improved with current therapies, and live birth rates of more than 80% can be achieved. However, some patients remain refractory and continue to have recurrent losses. Management of this group remains challenging; steroids, IVIG, and plasmapheresis have been tried with some benefit, but data are limited.[48–50] Therapy has to be individualized and the patient counseled accordingly.

Anti-Ro/La Antibodies and Neonatal Lupus Syndromes

Pregnancies exposed to anti-Ro and anti-La antibodies have higher risk of developing neonatal lupus syndromes (NLS), a form of passively acquired fetal autoimmunity from maternal antibodies that cross the placenta. Most manifestations, such as rash and hematologic and hepatic abnormalities, tend to resolve with clearance of the maternal antibodies by 6 to 8 months of life.[51] However, injury to the developing fetal cardiac conduction pathway by these antibodies can lead to permanent damage. The cardiac manifestations include conduction defects, structural abnormalities, cardiomyopathy, and congestive cardiac failure, but the most serious complication is development of complete heart block (CHB).[52]

Affecting up to 2% of exposed pregnancies, but with recurrence rates of 16% to 20% after the first event, CHB is associated with high fetal mortality of 20%. Most (up to 70%) survivors require pacemaker insertion.[53] CHB development is generally preceded by lower degrees of conduction delays, although rapid development without warning signs has been described.[53] Most events occur between 16 and 26 weeks of gestation but late cases do occur and even postpartum development of CHB has been reported. Early detection and treatment initiation might halt this progression but reversal of established CHB has not been reported. Multiple monitoring tools have been proposed for early detection of milder forms of conduction defects, including Doppler echocardiography, tissue velocity–based fetal kinetocardiogram, and transabdominal fetal electrocardiogram.[54]

Fetal Doppler echocardiography remains the most commonly used method. Based on the most vulnerable period, the recommended approach is to monitor all exposed fetuses weekly between 16 and 26 weeks of gestation, and biweekly thereafter.[52,55,56] Detection of an early conduction defect such as prolonged PR interval should prompt a discussion about prophylactic therapy. Although results have not been consistent, maternal administration of fluorinated corticosteroids and beta agonists has shown fetal survival benefit in some studies.[55,57–59] In the absence of any other therapy with known benefit, this remains the treatment of choice but any expected benefit has to be weighed against the risk of IUGR and preterm birth. Treatment of established CHB remains an unresolved issue with minimal benefit with any available approach.

The high risk of recurrence in subsequent pregnancies has prompted the quest for prophylactic therapy for at-risk pregnancies. Beneficial effects of IVIG were reported in open-label studies, but 2 large randomized controlled trials were negative.[60,61] Both trials have been criticized for methodology, and use of IVIG in this setting can still be considered as an option. However, the patient should be informed about the limited data and involved in the decision-making process.

HCQ again deserves special mention. Multiple studies have shown that HCQ reduces the risk of cardiac NLS in at-risk fetuses and possible recurrences.[62] In view of multiple beneficial effects of HCQ, need for continued use in all, and especially at-risk, pregnancies cannot be overemphasized.

Medication Use During Pregnancy

An important aspect of pregnancy management in SLE is optimization of medication use during this period. The choices of effective but safe immunosuppressants are discussed earlier.

The management of blood pressure can also become challenging because most of the antihypertensive drugs are contraindicated during pregnancy. The safe options include hydralazine, methyl-dopa, nifedipine, and labetalol.[63,64] β-Blocker use has been associated with IUGR and fetal bradycardia, and caution is required. Angiotensin-converting-enzyme inhibitors and angiotensin II receptor blockers are associated with specific malformations, neonatal arterial hypotension, and renal failure, and should be avoided.[63,65]

Nonsteroidal antiinflammatory drugs (NSAIDs) are generally considered safe during the first and second trimesters.[14] Recently, associations between NSAID use in the first trimester and specific birth defects were reported, along with potential risk of impaired fetal renal function with use after 20 weeks of gestation.[66] Hence, caution is required for use during early pregnancy. NSAIDs should be discontinued by 32 weeks of gestation in view of the significantly higher risk of premature closure of the ductus arteriosus. Cyclooxygenase 2 inhibitors should be avoided during pregnancy because data are very limited for safety evaluation.[14]

Antiplatelet agents considered safe for use during pregnancy include aspirin and clopidogrel.[67] However, clopidogrel has to be discontinued at least 7 days before delivery to avoid the increased risk of excessive hemorrhage. Heparin remains the anticoagulant of choice during pregnancy, with data emerging on the safety of the direct factor Xa inhibitor, fondoparinux.[67] LMWH is easier to use and has similar efficacy and safety to unfractionated heparin.[68] Warfarin is teratogenic and should be avoided during pregnancy, especially the first trimester.

Calcium supplementation is mandatory for all pregnant women with SLE, especially those receiving corticosteroids and heparin. Although low vitamin D levels during pregnancy have been associated with poor outcomes, supplemental vitamin D during pregnancy did not reduce the risk.[69,70] Bisphosphonates have long half-lives and use in women with reproductive potential should be carefully considered.

34. Vinet E, Pineau CA, Clarke AE, et al. Neurodevelopmental disorders in children born to mothers with systemic lupus erythematosus. Lupus 2014;23(11): 1099–104.

35. Chakravarty EF, Colon I, Langen ES, et al. Factors that predict prematurity and preeclampsia in pregnancies that are complicated by systemic lupus erythematosus. Am J Obstet Gynecol 2005;192(6):1897–904.

36. Hutcheon JA, Lisonkova S, Joseph KS. Epidemiology of pre-eclampsia and the other hypertensive disorders of pregnancy. Best Pract Res Clin Obstet Gynaecol 2011;25(4):391–403.

37. Salmon JE, Heuser C, Triebwasser M, et al. Mutations in complement regulatory proteins predispose to preeclampsia: a genetic analysis of the PROMISSE cohort. PLoS Med 2011;8(3):e1001013.

38. Kim MY, Buyon JP, Guerra MM, et al. Angiogenic factor imbalance early in pregnancy predicts adverse outcomes in patients with lupus and antiphospholipid antibodies: results of the PROMISSE study. Am J Obstet Gynecol 2016;214(1): 108.e1-14.

39. Kuc S, Wortelboer EJ, van Rijn BB, et al. Evaluation of 7 serum biomarkers and uterine artery Doppler ultrasound for first-trimester prediction of preeclampsia: a systematic review. Obstet Gynecol Surv 2011;66(4):225–39.

40. Kleinrouweler C, Wiegerinck M, Ris-Stalpers C, et al. Accuracy of circulating placental growth factor, vascular endothelial growth factor, soluble fms-like tyrosine kinase 1 and soluble endoglin in the prediction of pre-eclampsia: a systematic review and meta-analysis. BJOG 2012;119(7):778–87.

41. Chen TK, Gelber AC, Witter FR, et al. Renal biopsy in the management of lupus nephritis during pregnancy. Lupus 2015;24(2):147–54.

42. Yazdany J, Trupin L, Kaiser R, et al. Contraceptive counseling and use among women with systemic lupus erythematosus: a gap in health care quality? Arthritis Care Res (Hoboken) 2011;63(3):358–65.

43. Lateef A, Petri M. Hormone replacement and contraceptive therapy in autoimmune diseases. J Autoimmun 2012;38(2–3):J170–6.

44. Amengual O, Fujita D, Ota E, et al. Primary prophylaxis to prevent obstetric complications in asymptomatic women with antiphospholipid antibodies: a systematic review. Lupus 2015;24(11):1135–42.

45. Del Ross T, Ruffatti A, Visentin MS, et al. Treatment of 139 pregnancies in antiphospholipid-positive women not fulfilling criteria for antiphospholipid syndrome: a retrospective study. J Rheumatol 2013;40(4):425–9.

46. Empson M, Lassere M, Craig J, et al. Prevention of recurrent miscarriage for women with antiphospholipid antibody or lupus anticoagulant. Cochrane Database Syst Rev 2005;(2):CD002859.

47. Mak A, Cheung MW, Cheak AA, et al. Combination of heparin and aspirin is superior to aspirin alone in enhancing live births in patients with recurrent pregnancy loss and positive anti-phospholipid antibodies: a meta-analysis of randomized controlled trials and meta-regression. Rheumatology (Oxford) 2010;49(2):281–8.

48. Bramham K, Thomas M, Nelson-Piercy C, et al. First-trimester low-dose prednisolone in refractory antiphospholipid antibody-related pregnancy loss. Blood 2011;117(25):6948–51.

49. Branch DW, Peaceman AM, Druzin M, et al. A multicenter, placebo-controlled pilot study of intravenous immune globulin treatment of antiphospholipid syndrome during pregnancy. The Pregnancy Loss Study Group. Am J Obstet Gynecol 2000;182:122–7.

50. El-Haieg DO, Zanati MF, El-Foual FM. Plasmapheresis and pregnancy outcome in patients with antiphospholipid syndrome. Int J Gynaecol Obstet 2007;99(3): 236–41.

51. Izmirly PM, Rivera TL, Buyon JP. Neonatal lupus syndromes. Rheum Dis Clin North Am 2007;33(2):267–85, vi.

52. Brito-Zeron P, Izmirly PM, Ramos-Casals M, et al. The clinical spectrum of auto-immune congenital heart block. Nat Rev Rheumatol 2015;11(5):301–12.

53. Brito-Zeron P, Izmirly PM, Ramos-Casals M, et al. Autoimmune congenital heart block: complex and unusual situations. Lupus 2016;25(2):116–28.

54. Sonesson SE. Diagnosing foetal atrioventricular heart blocks. Scand J Immunol 2010;72(3):205–12.

55. Buyon JP, Clancy RM, Friedman DM. Cardiac manifestations of neonatal lupus erythematosus: guidelines to management, integrating clues from the bench and bedside. Nat Clin Pract Rheumatol 2009;5(3):139–48.

56. Friedman DM, Kim MY, Copel JA, et al. Prospective evaluation of fetuses with autoimmune-associated congenital heart block followed in the PR Interval and Dexamethasone Evaluation (PRIDE) Study. Am J Cardiol 2009;103(8):1102–6.

57. Levesque K, Morel N, Maltret A, et al. Description of 214 cases of autoimmune congenital heart block: results of the French neonatal lupus syndrome. Autoimmun Rev 2015;14(12):1154–60.

58. Izmirly PM, Saxena A, Sahl SK, et al. Assessment of fluorinated steroids to avert progression and mortality in anti-SSA/Ro-associated cardiac injury limited to the fetal conduction system. Ann Rheum Dis 2016;75(6):1161–5.

59. Jaeggi ET, Fouron JC, Silverman ED, et al. Transplacental fetal treatment improves the outcome of prenatally diagnosed complete atrioventricular block without structural heart disease. Circulation 2004;110(12):1542–8.

60. Friedman DM, Llanos C, Izmirly PM, et al. Evaluation of fetuses in a study of intravenous immunoglobulin as preventive therapy for congenital heart block: results of a multicenter, prospective, open-label clinical trial. Arthritis Rheum 2010;62(4): 1138–46.

61. Pisoni CN, Brucato A, Ruffatti A, et al. Failure of intravenous immunoglobulin to prevent congenital heart block: findings of a multicenter, prospective, observational study. Arthritis Rheum 2010;62(4):1147–52.

62. Peart E, Clowse ME. Systemic lupus erythematosus and pregnancy outcomes: an update and review of the literature. Curr Opin Rheumatol 2014;26(2):118–23.

63. American College of Obstetricians and Gynecologists. ACOG practice bulletin no. 125: chronic hypertension in pregnancy. Obstet Gynecol 2012;119(2 Pt 1): 396–407.

64. Mustafa R, Ahmed S, Gupta A, et al. A comprehensive review of hypertension in pregnancy. J Pregnancy 2012;2012:105918.

65. Cooper WO, Hernandez-Diaz S, Arbogast PG, et al. Major congenital malformations after first-trimester exposure to ACE inhibitors. N Engl J Med 2006;354(23): 2443–51.

66. Adams K, Bombardier C, van der Heijde DM. Safety of pain therapy during pregnancy and lactation in patients with inflammatory arthritis: a systematic literature review. J Rheumatol Suppl 2012;90:59–61.

67. Yarrington CD, Valente AM, Economy KE. Cardiovascular management in pregnancy: antithrombotic agents and antiplatelet agents. Circulation 2015;132(14): 1354–64.

68. Giannubilo SR, Tranquilli AL. Anticoagulant therapy during pregnancy for maternal and fetal acquired and inherited thrombophilia. Curr Med Chem 2012; 19(27):4562–71.
69. Aghajafari F, Nagulesapillai T, Ronksley PE, et al. Association between maternal serum 25-hydroxyvitamin D level and pregnancy and neonatal outcomes: systematic review and meta-analysis of observational studies. BMJ 2013;346:f1169.
70. De-Regil LM, Palacios C, Ansary A, et al. Vitamin D supplementation for women during pregnancy. Cochrane Database Syst Rev 2012;(2):CD008873.

Fertility, Pregnancy, and Lactation in Rheumatoid Arthritis

Pascal H.P. de Jong, MD, PhD, Radboud J.E.M. Dolhain, MD, PhD*

KEYWORDS

- Rheumatoid arthritis • Pregnancy • Fertility • Disease activity • Lactation

KEY POINTS

- Fertility is impaired in women with rheumatoid arthritis (RA), which is related to disease activity and the use of certain medications (nonsteroidal anti-inflammatory drugs and prednisone >7.5 mg daily).
- Although disease activity often improves in pregnancy, a substantial number of patients with RA still have active disease during pregnancy.
- Pregnancy outcomes in patients with RA are slightly less favorable compared with the general population, especially in patients with active disease.
- A treat-to-target strategy, aiming for low disease activity, is recommended for patients with RA who wish to conceive.
- Increasing evidence exists to suggest safety of tumor necrosis factor inhibitors in patients with RA who are pregnant or have a desire for pregnancy.

INTRODUCTION

Rheumatoid arthritis (RA) is a systemic autoimmune disease characterized by chronic inflammation of multiple joints. Approximately 1% of people in western countries suffer from RA. RA often affects women and men in the prime of their lives, which is the period wherein decisions about parenthood are made. In women with RA, however, it seems to be more difficult to conceive, as a result of the disease and/or treatment.[1–3]

During pregnancy, disease activity often improves, although less than previously thought. A substantial number of patients with RA still have active disease during pregnancy and so use of antirheumatic drugs may be unavoidable, especially given

Disclosure Statement: P.H.P. de Jong has nothing to disclose. R.J.E.M. Dolhain received unrestricted research grants from the Dutch Arthritis Association (Reumafonds), a noncommercial fund-raising organization, and from UCB Pharma BV.
Department of Rheumatology, Erasmus MC, Postbus 2040, Rotterdam 3000 CA, The Netherlands
* Corresponding author. Erasmus MC, Room Nb 852, Postbus 2040, Rotterdam 3000 CA, The Netherlands.
E-mail address: r.dolhain@erasmusmc.nl

rheumatic.theclinics.com

that active disease is negatively associated with pregnancy outcome. However, some drugs, including methotrexate, are known to be teratogenic during pregnancy; additionally, safety data on other medications during pregnancy are lacking. Nevertheless, more medications are compatible with pregnancy than previously appreciated. Therefore, this review considers fertility, pregnancy, and lactation issues in relation to RA (activity) and/or use of antirheumatic drugs.

FERTILITY
Female Perspective

Several studies indicate that family size is diminished in women with RA as a result of impaired fertility, which already may be present before the diagnosis of RA is made.[1–3] Women with RA experience more difficulties in conceiving, as indicated by a longer time to pregnancy (TTP). Previous studies showed that 25% to 42% of patients with RA did not conceive within 1 year.[4] For comparison, in the general population, the median prevalence of subfertility, defined as TTP of greater than 12 months, is 9%, with a range of 3.5% to 24.2% depending on the geographic area.[5]

Different factors might be associated with the impaired fertility. Earlier menopause has been reported in women with RA, and it has been postulated that these patients may have a smaller ovarian reserve.[6] This could explain both impaired fertility as well as earlier menopause. In early RA, the levels of serum anti-Müllerian hormone (AMH), a reliable biomarker for ovarian reserve, did not differ from healthy controls.[7] On the other hand, Henes and colleagues[8] showed that AMH levels are decreased in established RA, suggesting that ovarian reserve declines secondary to the RA disease process.

Personal choices, due to RA-related concerns, have been shown to be at least partially responsible for the smaller family size, but cannot account for the observed impaired fertility.[9] Disease activity, on the other hand, appears to contribute to impaired fertility. Brouwer and colleagues[4] showed that 67% of women with active disease (Disease Activity Score-28 [DAS28] >5.1) had a TTP of more than 1 year compared with 30% in women in remission (DAS28 <2.6).

Antirheumatic drugs also have been associated with increased TTP,[4,10] including nonsteroidal anti-inflammatory drugs (NSAIDs) and prednisone (in a dose >7.5 mg daily).[4] NSAIDs inhibit the production of prostaglandins, which play a role in ovulation and blastocyst implantation.[6] The effect of glucocorticoids on fertility is possibly due to (1) a transient suppression of the hypothalamic-pituitary-ovarian axis or (2) a direct effect on the ovarian function and/or endometrium.[11,12] It has been postulated that previous use of methotrexate (MTX) might impair fertility. The association between MTX and impaired fertility is mainly based on studies in oncology and animal models.[6] Recent studies, however, demonstrated that prior and short-term MTX treatment, respectively, did not affect the TTP and ovarian reserve.[4,7]

Another reason for the impaired fertility in patients with RA might be a result of a lower intercourse frequency.[6] These studies, however, were mainly conducted in postmenopausal patients with RA, and it is unclear whether this also applies to younger patients with RA with a desire to conceive.[6]

Male Perspective

Less is known about fertility problems and pregnancy outcomes in male patients with RA, because no good studies have been performed. Lower testosterone levels have been described in men with RA, but whether this results in lower fertility is not known.[13]

Additionally, literature about the effect of antirheumatic drugs on fertility are scarce. Sulfasalazine (SSZ) may cause oligospermia, reduce sperm motility, and increase abnormal sperm morphology.[14] Fortunately, drug withdrawal usually results in recovery of spermatogenesis after 2 months.[14]

The 3E (Evidence, Expertise, Exchange) initiative on the use of MTX recommends discontinuing MTX at least 3 months before a planned pregnancy, although underlying evidence for this is lacking.[15] Recent studies showed that paternal use of low-dose MTX was not associated with an increased risk of birth defects,[16,17] although an important limitation of these studies was the relatively small sample size. Although oligospermia and reversible sterility have been observed in case reports, low-dose MTX is not, in general, linked to poor semen quality and quantity.[18] It was initially thought that tumor necrosis factor (TNF) blockers decreased sperm quality, but more recent studies show no effect[19–21] and confirm that TNF blockers do not impair male fertility and/or increase the risk of adverse pregnancy outcomes.[19–21] Glucocorticoids and chronic use of NSAIDs may impair male fertility, but again, clinical studies are lacking.[22,23] In vitro studies suggest that chloroquine may negatively impair sperm motility, but no clinical data are available.[18]

PREGNANCY
Disease Activity

Given that disease activity is associated with TTP as well as pregnancy outcome in patients with RA, accurately determining RA disease activity in pregnancy is important. It is noteworthy that the erythrocyte sedimentation rate (ESR) is elevated in all pregnant women, due to increased circulating fibrinogen, plasma expansion, and decreased hemoglobin concentration.[24,25] In contrast, C-reactive protein (CRP) is only slightly influenced by pregnancy. Pregnancy might also influence the visual analogue scale (VAS) of global health.[26] Therefore, disease activity indices without an ESR and VAS are preferred during pregnancy.[24,27,28]

Disease activity improves in pregnancy, which is probably the reason why this physiologic phenomenon has been investigated so extensively.[27,29–33] Hench[30] was the first to describe this phenomenon in a small retrospective study in 1938. Between 1950 and 1995, multiple retrospective and a few prospective studies confirmed his initial observation and showed that 54% to 95% of pregnant patients with RA improved, with up to 39% achieving a state of remission.[10,32,34–46]

In the past 2 decades, multiple larger prospective studies have been conducted, documenting less disease improvement than previously described.[29,34] In the PARA study, De Man and colleagues[34] showed that 48% of 52 patients with initial DAS28–CRP $\geq$3.2 improved during pregnancy. Improvement was defined as having a good and/or moderate European League Against Rheumatism (EULAR) response. In the third trimester, approximately 50% of all pregnant patients with RA, including those with remission or low disease activity at the beginning of pregnancy, had active disease (DAS28 $\geq$3.2), whereas 27% of patients were in remission (DAS28 <2.6).[34]

These different improvement rates between the earlier and more recent studies are probably due to (1) the study design (ie, retrospective versus prospective); (2) patient selection, in that some of the earlier studies included only patients with active disease; and (3) the use of various definitions for improvement and remission. In addition, clinical and radiographic outcomes have improved enormously in the past 2 decades due to new therapeutic options and a treat-to-target approach, resulting in a larger proportion of patients with RA entering their pregnancy with low disease activity.

After delivery, there is an increased risk of a flare in disease activity. Postpartum exacerbations range between 62% and 90% in several retrospective studies.[30–33] In the prospective PARA cohort, a flare rate after delivery was 39% despite restarting medication.[34,35] Interestingly, one-third of patients experience a flare of their disease activity after miscarriage as well.[34–36]

The pregnancy-associated improvement and postpartum exacerbation of RA are likely the result of multiple hormonal and immunologic changes during pregnancy followed by the gradual return of these changes to prepregnancy values after delivery.[37] Although multiple factors have been investigated, the exact mechanisms underlying these phenomena remain unknown.

Pregnancy Outcome

Pregnancy outcome in patients with RA is slightly less favorable, especially in patients with active disease, when compared with the general population.[38–41] Brouwer and colleagues[36] showed that the risk of a miscarriage in women with RA (17%) is comparable to the general population (11%–22%). The investigators suggest that this miscarriage rate in patients with RA might be an underestimation, however, for the following reasons: (1) the investigated cohort consisted of patients with RA with a planned pregnancy and therefore did not use MTX, which is associated with an increased risk of miscarriage; and (2) there were fewer smokers and more patients with higher education levels in this cohort than in the general population.[36]

Recently, Wallenius and colleagues[42] confirmed concerns regarding miscarriage risk within a Norwegian birth registry, and showed a slightly increased miscarriage rate in women with RA compared with women without an inflammatory disease, with an odds ratio (95% confidence interval) of 1.32 (1.19–1.47).

Preeclampsia is a relatively uncommon pregnancy complication. Using a large population-based health care registry, Norgaard and colleagues[39] showed that the risk of preeclampsia increased slightly from 3.4% in unaffected women to 5.0% in women with RA and a first-time singleton birth. Other studies did not confirm the previous finding, however, probably the result of a lack of power.[43]

Pregnant patients with RA have an increased risk for a Cesarean delivery (26%–34%) when compared with the general population (16.5%–19.5%).[39,44] De Man and colleagues[43] showed that active disease was associated with an increased risk for Cesarean delivery: 22% for the active disease group (DAS28–CRP $\geq$3.2) versus 10% in the group with less active disease (DAS28–CRP <3.2). However, data on Cesarean delivery should be interpreted with caution, as indications to perform a Cesarean delivery may vary for different countries.

The risk of preterm delivery, defined as a birth before 37 weeks of gestation, is increased in women with RA (9.2%–15.2%) compared with healthy controls (6.2%–7.8%).[38,39,44,45] Factors associated with preterm delivery are disease severity and the use of glucocorticoids.[41,43]

Impact for the Child

There is no increased risk of major congenital malformations or perinatal death found in children born to women with RA.[44,45] However, multiple studies report on increased risk of small-for-gestational-age (SGA) infants in women with RA (~10%) compared with healthy controls (~3%).[38–41,45] De Man and colleagues[43] demonstrated that an increase in RA disease activity during pregnancy is independently associated with lower birth weight in the offspring, although still within the normal range. In this study, the incidence of SGA infants was 3.3%.[43]

Lower birth weight (even within the normal range) has been associated with an increased risk of cardiovascular and metabolic disease in adulthood.[46,47] This effect is even more prominent if the children display rapid catch-up growth in weight during their first year of life. A recent study showed that 28% of children born to women with

RA show rapid catch-up growth, and this was associated with maternal disease activity.[48] However, when these children were reevaluated at age 7, they did not have a high-risk profile in anthropometric measures, such as an increased blood pressure or altered body composition compared with healthy controls.[49]

ANTIRHEUMATIC DRUGS DURING PREGNANCY AND LACTATION

Recently, the EULAR published "points to consider" for the use of antirheumatic drugs during pregnancy and lactation.[50] Following we summarize current recommendations and additional background information when needed (**Table 1**).

Table 1
Use of disease-modifying agents during pregnancy and lactation

Medication	Pregnancy	Lactation
Nonsteroidal anti-inflammatory drugs	May impair fertility Stop before 32 wk gestation (premature closure of ductus arteriosus)	Low concentrations in breast milk Compatible with breastfeeding
Glucocorticoids	Nonfluorinated glucocorticoid (prednisone) metabolized by the placenta Compatible with pregnancy Use lowest dose for the shortest duration necessary	Compatible with breastfeeding
Methotrexate	Known teratogen Discontinue 3 mo before pregnancy	Can be detected in breast milk
Leflunomide	Teratogenic in animal studies Small human studies show no increased risks Cholestyramine washout before pregnancy strongly recommended	Limited data on breastfeeding Avoid use during breastfeeding
Sulfasalazine	Compatible with pregnancy at doses ≤2 g daily Folate supplementation strongly recommended	Compatible with breastfeeding full-term infants Avoid use in premature or ill infants
Hydroxychloroquine	Compatible with pregnancy	Compatible with breastfeeding
Tumor necrosis factor inhibitors	Actively crosses placenta during second trimester Most studies found no increased risk of birth defects Low placental transfer of etanercept and certolizumab throughout pregnancy Postpone live vaccines in exposed infants for 6 mo	Compatible with breastfeeding
Other biologicals	Limited human data on pregnancy exposure Recommend avoiding during pregnancy	Limited data on breastfeeding Avoid use during breastfeeding

Nonsteroidal Anti-inflammatory Drugs

NSAIDs are associated with a longer TTP.[6] First-trimester and second-trimester exposure to NSAIDs is not teratogenic. After 20 weeks of gestation, NSAIDs can impair renal function and may cause constriction of the ductus arteriosus, which increases with gestational age. In addition, NSAIDs impair labor; therefore, NSAIDs should be stopped before the 32nd gestational week. Data on the safety of cyclooxygenase-2 inhibitors are scarce and so it is sometimes recommended to switch to traditional NSAIDs during pregnancy.[51]

NSAIDs can be detected only in very low concentrations in breast milk and are considered compatible with breastfeeding.[50]

Glucocorticoids

Nonfluorinated glucocorticoids, such as prednisone, are largely metabolized by the placenta, and, as a result, less than 10% of the drug reaches the fetus. In general, nonfluorinated glucocorticoids are not considered to be teratogenic.[51,52] On the other hand, the use of glucocorticoids is associated with intrauterine growth restriction, shorter gestational age, and premature rupture of the membranes,[4,51,52] so both dose and duration of glucocorticoid should be minimized.

Fluorinated glucocorticoids are not metabolized by the placenta and should, therefore, be restricted to fetal indications.[51] Glucocorticoids are compatible with breastfeeding.[50]

Disease-Modifying Antirheumatic Drugs

MTX is teratogenic and induces miscarriages and should be avoided during pregnancy.[51,53] In general, it is advised to stop MTX 3 months before a planned pregnancy.[15] MTX can be detected in small amounts in breast milk and should be not be taken while breastfeeding because of theoretic risk.[51]

Leflunomide is teratogenic in animal studies. Some human studies, however, reported no increased risk of congenital malformations after first-trimester exposure to leflunomide, when followed by cholestyramine washout.[51] Due to limited data, it is recommended that leflunomide be avoided during pregnancy; however, with a washout procedure before pregnancy attempts, according to current expert opinion.[50] Data on leflunomide and breast feeding are scarce and should, therefore, be avoided in lactating women.[50]

Several studies have shown that sulfasalazine (SSZ), in a dose ≤2 g daily, can be used safely during pregnancy, even though SSZ does cross the placenta.[51] SSZ inhibits the gastrointestinal and cellular uptake of folate and, therefore, folate supplementation should be prescribed throughout pregnancy. SSZ has been found in very low concentrations in breast milk, but concentrations of sulfapyridine, a metabolite of SSZ, can range between 30% and 60% of maternal serum levels. Nevertheless, breastfeeding is considered safe in the healthy, full-term infant.[50] SSZ should be avoided in lactating women, however, if their newborn has one of following conditions: dysmaturity, prematurity, hyperbilirubinemia, ill health, or a glucose-6-phosphate dehydrogenase deficiency.[51]

Hydroxychloroquine crosses the placenta, but no increase in congenital malformations was reported in several hundreds of pregnancies at the recommended daily dose of 200 to 400 mg. Moreover, long-term follow-up studies of children have not revealed visual, hearing, or developmental abnormalities.[50,51] Hydroxychloroquine can be detected in only trace amounts in breast milk and is, therefore, considered compatible with breastfeeding.[50,51]

Azathioprine and cyclosporine are considered safe during pregnancy, but they are rarely prescribed during pregnancy for RA because of a less favorable benefit-risk balance.[51]

Tumor Necrosis Factor Blockers

Increasingly more data are available on the use of TNF blockers during pregnancy. Most data are for infliximab and adalimumab, followed by etanercept and certolizumab, and there are limited data on golimumab. Recently, a large prospective study showed a small increase in major birth defects after exposure to TNF blockers during the first trimester with odds ratio (95% confidence interval) of 2.20 (1.0–4.8). However, no distinct pattern of malformations could be identified and the birth defect rate in the healthy controls of that study was lower than in the general population (2.2%).[54] Furthermore, other studies have not found an association between the use of TNF blockers and congenital abnormalities or adverse pregnancy outcomes.[55]

TNF inhibitors that contain an Fc part of an immunoglobulin G molecule are actively transported from the maternal to the fetal circulation starting at approximately week 18 of gestation.[56] After third-trimester exposure to infliximab and adalimumab, serum levels can be up to 3 times higher in the newborn compared with the mother and may still be detected 6 months after birth.[57] Placental transport may be less of a concern for etanercept and certolizumab.[57,58] Because of the aforementioned issues, it is advisable to postpone all live vaccines for the infant until 6 months of age after exposure to TNF blockers in the third trimester, with the exception of certolizumab.[59]

Recently published EULAR recommendations advise considering continuation of TNF blockers during the first part of pregnancy.[50] Etanercept and certolizumab may even be considered for use throughout pregnancy due to low rates of transplacental passage.[50]

TNF blockers are compatible with breastfeeding, because minimal transfer to breast milk has been shown, for infliximab, adalimumab, etanercept, and certolizumab.[50]

Other Biologicals

Tocilizumab, abatacept, rituximab, and anakinra are other biologicals used for the treatment of RA. Limited or no data on the safe use in pregnancy or during lactation are available on the aforementioned biologicals and these biologicals should, therefore, be avoided in pregnancy and during lactation.[50]

SUMMARY

Fertility is impaired in women with RA, related to both disease activity and the use of certain medication (NSAIDs and prednisone >7.5 mg daily). Less is known about fertility problems in men with RA.

Although disease activity often improves in pregnancy, a substantial number of patients with RA (>50%) will still have active disease during pregnancy. Pregnancy outcomes in patients with RA are slightly less favorable when compared with the general population, especially in those patients with active disease. Therefore, a treat-to-target strategy aiming for low disease activity is recommended for patients with RA who wish to conceive.

Controlling RA disease activity during pregnancy is challenging, especially because several antirheumatic drugs are contraindicated in pregnancy. Still, many more treatment options are available than in the past. Increasing evidence on the safe use of TNF inhibitors in pregnant patients with RA is available, particularly during the first trimester and early second trimester. As a result, several TNF blockers can be continued up to a certain gestational age, according to the recently published EULAR recommendations.

REFERENCES

1. Wallenius M, Skomsvoll JF, Irgens LM, et al. Fertility in women with chronic inflammatory arthritides. Rheumatology (Oxford) 2011;50(6):1162–7.
2. Wallenius M, Skomsvoll JF, Irgens LM, et al. Parity in patients with chronic inflammatory arthritides childless at time of diagnosis. Scand J Rheumatol 2012;41(3): 202–7.
3. Skomsvoll JF, Ostensen M, Baste V, et al. Number of births, interpregnancy interval, and subsequent pregnancy rate after a diagnosis of inflammatory rheumatic disease in Norwegian women. J Rheumatol 2001;28(10):2310–4.
4. Brouwer J, Hazes JM, Laven JS, et al. Fertility in women with rheumatoid arthritis: influence of disease activity and medication. Ann Rheum Dis 2015;74(10): 1836–41.
5. Boivin J, Bunting L, Collins JA, et al. International estimates of infertility prevalence and treatment-seeking: potential need and demand for infertility medical care. Hum Reprod 2007;22(6):1506–12.
6. Provost M, Eaton JL, Clowse ME. Fertility and infertility in rheumatoid arthritis. Curr Opin Rheumatol 2014;26(3):308–14.
7. Brouwer J, Laven JS, Hazes JM, et al. Levels of serum anti-Mullerian hormone, a marker for ovarian reserve, in women with rheumatoid arthritis. Arthritis Care Res (Hoboken) 2013;65(9):1534–8.
8. Henes M, Froeschlin J, Taran FA, et al. Ovarian reserve alterations in premenopausal women with chronic inflammatory rheumatic diseases: impact of rheumatoid arthritis, Behcet's disease and spondyloarthritis on anti-Mullerian hormone levels. Rheumatology (Oxford) 2015;54(9):1709–12.
9. Clowse ME, Chakravarty E, Costenbader KH, et al. Effects of infertility, pregnancy loss, and patient concerns on family size of women with rheumatoid arthritis and systemic lupus erythematosus. Arthritis Care Res (Hoboken) 2012;64(5):668–74.
10. Ince-Askan H, Dolhain RJ. Pregnancy and rheumatoid arthritis. Best Pract Res Clin Rheumatol 2015;29(4–5):580–96.
11. Saketos M, Sharma N, Santoro NF. Suppression of the hypothalamic-pituitary-ovarian axis in normal women by glucocorticoids. Biol Reprod 1993;49(6): 1270–6.
12. Whirledge S, Cidlowski JA. A role for glucocorticoids in stress-impaired reproduction: beyond the hypothalamus and pituitary. Endocrinology 2013;154(12): 4450–68.
13. Gordon D, Beastall GH, Thomson JA, et al. Androgenic status and sexual function in males with rheumatoid arthritis and ankylosing spondylitis. Q J Med 1986;60(231):671–9.
14. O'Morain C, Smethurst P, Dore CJ, et al. Reversible male infertility due to sulphasalazine: studies in man and rat. Gut 1984;25(10):1078–84.
15. Visser K, Katchamart W, Loza E, et al. Multinational evidence-based recommendations for the use of methotrexate in rheumatic disorders with a focus on rheumatoid arthritis: integrating systematic literature research and expert opinion of a broad international panel of rheumatologists in the 3E initiative. Ann Rheum Dis 2009;68(7):1086–93.

16. Wallenius M, Lie E, Daltveit AK, et al. No excess risks in offspring with paternal preconception exposure to disease-modifying antirheumatic drugs. Arthritis Rheumatol 2015;67(1):296–301.

17. Weber-Schoendorfer C, Hoeltzenbein M, Wacker E, et al. No evidence for an increased risk of adverse pregnancy outcome after paternal low-dose methotrexate: an observational cohort study. Rheumatology (Oxford) 2014;53(4): 757–63.

18. Millsop JW, Heller MM, Eliason MJ, et al. Dermatological medication effects on male fertility. Dermatol Ther 2013;26(4):337–46.

19. Puchner R, Danninger K, Puchner A, et al. Impact of TNF-blocking agents on male sperm characteristics and pregnancy outcomes in fathers exposed to TNF-blocking agents at time of conception. Clin Exp Rheumatol 2012;30(5): 765–7.

20. Ramonda R, Foresta C, Ortolan A, et al. Influence of tumor necrosis factor alpha inhibitors on testicular function and semen in spondyloarthritis patients. Fertil Steril 2014;101(2):359–65.

21. Micu MC, Micu R, Surd S, et al. TNF-alpha inhibitors do not impair sperm quality in males with ankylosing spondylitis after short-term or long-term treatment. Rheumatology (Oxford) 2014;53(7):1250–5.

22. Whirledge S, Cidlowski JA. Glucocorticoids, stress, and fertility. Minerva Endocrinol 2010;35(2):109–25.

23. Martini AC, Molina RI, Tissera AD, et al. Analysis of semen from patients chronically treated with low or moderate doses of aspirin-like drugs. Fertil Steril 2003; 80(1):221–2.

24. de Man YA, Hazes JM, van de Geijn FE, et al. Measuring disease activity and functionality during pregnancy in patients with rheumatoid arthritis. Arthritis Rheum 2007;57(5):716–22.

25. van den Broe NR, Letsky EA. Pregnancy and the erythrocyte sedimentation rate. BJOG 2001;108(11):1164–7.

26. Prevoo ML, van 't Hof MA, Kuper HH, et al. Modified disease activity scores that include twenty-eight-joint counts. Development and validation in a prospective longitudinal study of patients with rheumatoid arthritis. Arthritis Rheum 1995; 38(1):44–8.

27. Ostensen M, Husby G. A prospective clinical study of the effect of pregnancy on rheumatoid arthritis and ankylosing spondylitis. Arthritis Rheum 1983;26(9): 1155–9.

28. de Man YA, Dolhain RJ, Hazes JM. Disease activity or remission of rheumatoid arthritis before, during and following pregnancy. Curr Opin Rheumatol 2014; 26(3):329–33.

29. Barrett JH, Brennan P, Fiddler M, et al. Does rheumatoid arthritis remit during pregnancy and relapse postpartum? Results from a nationwide study in the United Kingdom performed prospectively from late pregnancy. Arthritis Rheum 1999;42(6):1219–27.

30. Hench PS. The ameliorating effect of pregnancy on chronic atrophic (infectious rheumatoid) arthritis, fibrositis and intermittent hydrarthritis. Mayo Clin Proc 1938;13:7.

31. Oka M. Effect of pregnancy on the onset and course of rheumatoid arthritis. Ann Rheum Dis 1953;12(3):227–9.

32. Ostensen M, Aune B, Husby G. Effect of pregnancy and hormonal changes on the activity of rheumatoid arthritis. Scand J Rheumatol 1983;12(2):69–72.

33. Klipple GL, Cecere FA. Rheumatoid arthritis and pregnancy. Rheum Dis Clin North Am 1989;15(2):213–39.

34. de Man YA, Dolhain RJ, van de Geijn FE, et al. Disease activity of rheumatoid arthritis during pregnancy: results from a nationwide prospective study. Arthritis Rheum 2008;59(9):1241–8.

35. de Man YA, Bakker-Jonges LE, Goorbergh CM, et al. Women with rheumatoid arthritis negative for anti-cyclic citrullinated peptide and rheumatoid factor are more likely to improve during pregnancy, whereas in autoantibody-positive women autoantibody levels are not influenced by pregnancy. Ann Rheum Dis 2010;69(2):420–3.

36. Brouwer J, Laven JS, Hazes JM, et al. Brief report: miscarriages in female rheumatoid arthritis patients: associations with serologic findings, disease activity, and antirheumatic drug treatment. Arthritis Rheumatol 2015;67(7):1738–43.

37. Ostensen M, Villiger PM. The remission of rheumatoid arthritis during pregnancy. Semin Immunopathol 2007;29(2):185–91.

38. Skomsvoll JF, Ostensen M, Irgens LM, et al. Perinatal outcome in pregnancies of women with connective tissue disease and inflammatory rheumatic disease in Norway. Scand J Rheumatol 1999;28(6):352–6.

39. Norgaard M, Larsson H, Pedersen L, et al. Rheumatoid arthritis and birth outcomes: a Danish and Swedish nationwide prevalence study. J Intern Med 2010;268(4):329–37.

40. Lin HC, Chen SF, Chen YH. Increased risk of adverse pregnancy outcomes in women with rheumatoid arthritis: a nationwide population-based study. Ann Rheum Dis 2010;69(4):715–7.

41. Bharti B, Lee SJ, Lindsay SP, et al. Disease severity and pregnancy outcomes in women with rheumatoid arthritis: results from the organization of teratology information specialists autoimmune diseases in pregnancy project. J Rheumatol 2015;42(8):1376–82.

42. Wallenius M, Salvesen KA, Daltveit AK, et al. Miscarriage and stillbirth in women with rheumatoid arthritis. J Rheumatol 2015;42(9):1570–2.

43. de Man YA, Hazes JM, van der Heide H, et al. Association of higher rheumatoid arthritis disease activity during pregnancy with lower birth weight: results of a national prospective study. Arthritis Rheum 2009;60(11):3196–206.

44. Reed SD, Vollan TA, Svec MA. Pregnancy outcomes in women with rheumatoid arthritis in Washington state. Matern Child Health J 2006;10(4):361–6.

45. Wolfberg AJ, Lee-Parritz A, Peller AJ, et al. Association of rheumatologic disease with preeclampsia. Obstet Gynecol 2004;103(6):1190–3.

46. Ong KK, Dunger DB. Perinatal growth failure: the road to obesity, insulin resistance and cardiovascular disease in adults. Best Pract Res Clin Endocrinol Metab 2002;16(2):191–207.

47. Leunissen RW, Kerkhof GF, Stijnen T, et al. Timing and tempo of first-year rapid growth in relation to cardiovascular and metabolic risk profile in early adulthood. JAMA 2009;301(21):2234–42.

48. de Steenwinkel FD, Hokken-Koelega AC, de Ridder MA, et al. Rheumatoid arthritis during pregnancy and postnatal catch-up growth in the offspring. Arthritis Rheumatol 2014;66(7):1705–11.

49. de Steenwinkel FDO, Dolhain REJM, Hazes JMW, et al. Does elevated disease activity or medication use influence the body composition of the prepubertal offspring in pregnant women with rheumatoid arthritis? Arthritis Rheum 2013; 65:1.

50. Gotestam Skorpen C, Hoeltzenbein M, Tincani A, et al. The EULAR points to consider for use of antirheumatic drugs before pregnancy, and during pregnancy and lactation. Ann Rheum Dis 2016;75(5):795–810.
51. Ostensen M, Khamashta M, Lockshin M, et al. Anti-inflammatory and immunosuppressive drugs and reproduction. Arthritis Res Ther 2006;8(3):209.
52. Bermas BL. Non-steroidal anti inflammatory drugs, glucocorticoids and disease modifying anti-rheumatic drugs for the management of rheumatoid arthritis before and during pregnancy. Curr Opin Rheumatol 2014;26(3):334–40.
53. Weber-Schoendorfer C, Chambers C, Wacker E, et al. Pregnancy outcome after methotrexate treatment for rheumatic disease prior to or during early pregnancy: a prospective multicenter cohort study. Arthritis Rheumatol 2014;66(5):1101–10.
54. Weber-Schoendorfer C, Oppermann M, Wacker E, et al. Pregnancy outcome after TNF-alpha inhibitor therapy during the first trimester: a prospective multicentre cohort study. Br J Clin Pharmacol 2015;80(4):727–39.
55. Chaudrey KH, Kane SV. Safety of immunomodulators and anti-TNF therapy in pregnancy. Curr Treat Options Gastroenterol 2015;13(1):77–89.
56. Malek A, Sager R, Kuhn P, et al. Evolution of maternofetal transport of immunoglobulins during human pregnancy. Am J Reprod Immunol 1996;36(5):248–55.
57. Mahadevan U, Wolf DC, Dubinsky M, et al. Placental transfer of anti-tumor necrosis factor agents in pregnant patients with inflammatory bowel disease. Clin Gastroenterol Hepatol 2013;11(3):286–92 [quiz: e224].
58. Berthelsen BG, Fjeldsoe-Nielsen H, Nielsen CT, et al. Etanercept concentrations in maternal serum, umbilical cord serum, breast milk and child serum during breastfeeding. Rheumatology (Oxford) 2010;49(11):2225–7.
59. Hyrich KL, Verstappen SM. Biologic therapies and pregnancy: the story so far. Rheumatology (Oxford) 2014;53(8):1377–85.

Vasculitis and Pregnancy

Leah Machen, MD[a], Megan E.B. Clowse, MD, MPH[b],*

KEYWORDS

- Vasculitis • Pregnancy • Prednisone • TNF-Inhibitor • ANCA-associated vasculitis
- Behçet disease • Takayasu arteritis

KEY POINTS

- There are limited data to guide the management of vasculitis during pregnancy.
- Pregnancies that occur when vasculitis is well controlled and on medications considered low risk will result in the best opportunity for success.
- Although cyclophosphamide, methotrexate, and mycophenolate mofetil are known to cause pregnancy loss and congenital anomalies, the other medications that are typically used for vasculitis are largely considered low risk.

INTRODUCTION

Vasculitis is more often a disease affecting women beyond their reproductive years, making the challenges of pregnancy management difficult to study. Improved diagnostic capabilities and treatment options have both prolonged patient survival and led to earlier age of diagnosis, which in turn has increased the number of pregnancies in this population. Because of the earlier median age of onset in Behçet disease (BD) and Takayasu arteritis (TA), most of the literature focuses on pregnancies in women with these diseases; however, cases of pregnancy during antineutrophil cytoplasmic antibody (ANCA)–associated vasculitis have also been reported in the literature.[1] The various physiologic changes of pregnancy may have both positive and negative impacts on maternal vasculitis. Hormonal and endocrine changes during pregnancy may alter cytokines favoring the Th2-cytokine polarization, allowing a worsening of Th2-cytokine–mediated diseases, such as ANCA-associated vasculitis, and improving Th1-cytokine–mediated disorders, such as BD and TA.[2] However, when carefully timed and managed, most pregnancies in patients with systemic vasculitis can be successful with minimal antepartum complications and minimal impact on disease process.

Disclosure: Neither author has any commercial or financial conflicts to report. No funding sources.
[a] Department of Medicine, Duke University Medical Center, Durham, NC, USA; [b] Division of Rheumatology, Duke University Medical Center, Box 3535 Trent Drive, Durham, NC 27710, USA
* Corresponding author.
E-mail address: megan.clowse@duke.edu

ANTINEUTROPHIL CYTOPLASMIC ANTIBODY–ASSOCIATED VASCULITIS, INCLUDING GRANULOMATOSIS WITH POLYANGIITIS, MICROSCOPIC POLYANGIITIS, AND EOSINOPHILIC GRANULOMATOSIS WITH POLYANGIITIS

ANCA-associated vasculitis includes granulomatosis with polyangiitis (GPA, formerly Wegener granulomatosis), microscopic polyangiitis (MPA), and eosinophilic granulomatosis with polyangiitis (EGPA, formerly Churg Strauss). Although the prevalence of these diseases is relatively low in women of childbearing age because the mean age of onset is later in life, there are documented cases of pregnancies for each of these forms of ANCA-associated vasculitis.

Effect of Antineutrophil Cytoplasmic Antibody–Associated Vasculitis on Pregnancy

GPA is a necrotizing vasculitis that typically affects the upper respiratory tract, lungs, and kidney with a peak age of onset after 40 years.[2] MPA is a small vessel, necrotizing, pauci-immune vasculitis with complications, including severe renal disease and pulmonary hemorrhage.[3] Preterm delivery is a common complication of GPA with rates as high as 35%, particularly when the disease is active during pregnancy.[4,5] Preeclampsia, premature rupture of membranes, spontaneous abortion, prepartum hemorrhage, and retroplacental hematoma have all been reported.[6,7] Poorer outcomes are associated with women who conceived with active disease or who had onset of GPA during pregnancy.[8] There are limited data on the effects of MPA on pregnancy and vice versa, primarily consisting of case reports. In the few cases that have been reported, complications included maternal death,[9] low birth weight,[10] prematurity, and the occurrence of an MPA-like syndrome in the newborn.[11]

EGPA is characterized by extravascular necrotizing granulomas rich in eosinophils, peripheral blood eosinophilia, and pulmonary and small vessel vasculitis occurring in patients with asthma and allergic rhinitis.[3] The mean age of disease onset is approximately 48 years. As with GPA, preterm birth was the most common complication of pregnancy; however, fetal loss, intrauterine growth restriction (IUGR), and cesarean delivery were also observed.[12]

Effect of Pregnancy on Antineutrophil Cytoplasmic Antibody–Associated Vasculitis

With all forms of systemic vasculitis, complications are most severe and outcomes most devastating if pregnancy occurs during a disease flare.[6] This point holds true for ANCA-associated vasculitis: high levels of disease activity persisted throughout pregnancy in most women who became pregnant with active disease; however, only 40% of those who conceived while in remission developed a disease flare.[3] GPA flares during pregnancy mostly consisted of respiratory complications, subglottic stenosis, skin lesions, arthritis, and renal deterioration. However, it can be difficult to differentiate renal impairment from GPA flare or preeclampsia.[13,14]

Vasculitis complications were also seen in cases of EGPA with complications as severe as maternal death.[15,16] Complications were reported in patients with MPA also, with most symptoms involving rash, joint swelling, pain, and fever.[12] The frequency of these complications is difficult to extrapolate to the general population considering the scarce data available.

Although the numbers are limited, ANCA-associated vasculitis seems to be more frequently reported to start during pregnancy than most other rheumatic diseases.[3] Based on the available data, it is not possible to assess whether established ANCA-associated vasculitis flares more often during pregnancy than other autoimmune disorders. In a patient-reported retrospective study, only 20% of patients reported a vasculitis flare during pregnancy.[17] In small prospective cohorts followed in university centers, however, vasculitis flare during pregnancy seems to be more common **(Table 1)**.[7]

Table 1 A summary of published data about antineutrophil cytoplasmic antibody–associated vasculitis in pregnancy				
Study	Number of Pregnancies	Pregnancy Loss	Preterm Birth	Vasculitis Activity During Pregnancy
Gatto et al,[3] 2012	48	4 (8%)	17 (35%)	15 (45%)
Pagnoux et al,[7] 2011	22	6 (27%)	8 (36%)	2 (Major flare)[a]
Fredi et al,[18] 2015	17	1 (5%)	4 (23%)	6 (35%)

[a] One patient with acute cardiac decompensation and another with rupture of pancreatic microaneurysm.

POLYARTERITIS NODOSA

Polyarteritis nodosa (PAN) is a disorder characterized by necrotizing inflammation of medium size or small arteries, with prevalent features of musculoskeletal, gastrointestinal (GI), and neuropathic involvement. Pregnancy outcomes are generally favorable with rare disease relapse and the birth of healthy babies when patients conceive during disease remission. Reported complications include preterm delivery and IUGR. However, consequences of conceiving during active PAN, and particularly development of a new diagnosis during pregnancy, can be devastating. In 2 reports from the 1980s, 7 out of 8 patients with onset of PAN during pregnancy died during gestation or within the first 2 months of delivery; in many of these cases, the diagnosis was made post mortem.[19,20]

TAKAYASU ARTERITIS

TA is a granulomatous vasculitis that affects large vessels including the aorta and its branches. TA frequently presents in the second or third decade of life and is more commonly observed in pregnancy than other forms of vasculitis because of the earlier age of onset.[3,21]

Effect of Takayasu Arteritis on Pregnancy

Most pregnancies in patients with TA are successful; however, women with TA are predisposed to complications, particularly during the peripartum period. Severe HTN and preeclampsia are the most frequent complications of pregnancy in women with TA, with a prevalence of approximately 40% in patients with TA compared with 8% in the general population. Intrauterine fetal death may also be more common in TA.[22–24] In a recent systematic review of more than 200 pregnancies in women with TA, up to 20% of pregnancies were complicated by either IUGR or low birth weight **(Table 2)**.[3] Other complications included preterm delivery and fetal loss, with risk of maternal and fetal complications greater in patients with more severe maternal disease.[25] Patients with renal artery and abdominal aorta involvement experienced more frequent complications of preeclampsia and IUGR.[25]

Because of proximal stenosis causing occult central hypertension (HTN), some groups suggest elective cesarean deliveries in order to avoid the straining of labor, thus, increasing the rate of cesarean birth in this population.[18] Although there are not currently adequate data to dictate the best approach to delivery for this population, the obstetric and anesthesia teams should be aware of the hypertensive risk and use of aggressive hemodynamic monitoring may be indicated.

Effect of Pregnancy on Takayasu Arteritis

Recent studies have shown that pregnancy does not have a significant effect on TA in most cases; however, if complications do occur, implications can be severe. Maternal complications such as development of aortic aneurysm, stroke, congestive heart failure, aortic insufficiency, myocardial infarction, and aortic dissection are rare but devastating.[26–31] Aortic dissection can occur during pregnancy in women with TA, suggesting that chest pain in this population be urgently and fully evaluated.[32] More common complications include progression of renal insufficiency, anemia, thrombocytopenia, and elevated inflammatory markers.[25,26]

Table 2
A summary of published data about Takayasu arteritis in pregnancy

Study	Number of Pregnancies	Pregnancy Loss[a]	Preterm Delivery	TA Complications[b]	Treatment Information
Gatto et al,[3] 2012	214	40 (18.6%)	35 (16%)	25 (11.6%)	Recommends treatment with corticosteroids for disease relapse during pregnancy and azathioprine for refractory cases
Assad et al,[33] 2015	156	20 (12.8%)	28 (17.9%)	9 (5.8%)	Showed no association between maternal/fetal outcomes with steroid use
Comarmond et al,[34] 2015	98	12 (12.2%)	8 (8.2%)	38 (38.8%)	No significant difference in maternal complications with anti–IL-6 therapy or corticosteroids but noted a trend implying patients receiving therapy have fewer complications

Abbreviation: IL-6, interleukin 6.
   [a] Including medical termination.
   [b] Maternal complications and disease flares,[3] carotidynia, fever,[33] worsening hypertension, arterial stenosis/occlusion, pulmonary embolism, aortic aneurysm, stroke, renal failure, infection.

BEHÇET DISEASE

BD is a chronic relapsing inflammatory disease with recurrent oral and genital ulcers, ocular and GI manifestations, and thrombosis.[35] It mostly affects young women of childbearing age; thus, it represents a significant proportion of systemic vasculitis data worldwide.

Effect of Behçet Disease on Pregnancy

Based on data from more than 225 pregnancies in women with BD, it seems that pregnancy outcomes are fairly similar to those seen in the general population (**Table 3**).[3] A case-control study in 2005 reported higher frequencies of preterm birth and pregnancy loss among women with BD compared with healthy women, but the absolute rates were within what is expected normally.[36] Complications of spontaneous abortion, IUGR, premature deliveries, gestational diabetes, and HTN have also been reported.[36–38]

Effects of Pregnancy on Behçet Disease

In approximately 60% of cases, BD improves or remains stable during pregnancy; however, 30% of patients experience relapse consisting primarily of ulceration, arthritis, uveitis, erythema nodosum, and, infrequently, thrombosis.[3] In a systematic review, thrombotic events were reported in 6 patients (3%).[3] Pregnancy is a period of hypercoagulability for all women, possibly compounding the risk for women with BD who are prone to clotting. Patients with prior thrombosis should be strongly considered as candidates for anticoagulation during pregnancy.

Table 3
A summary of published data about Behçet disease in pregnancy

Article	Number of Pregnancies	Pregnancy Loss	Preterm Delivery	BD Complications	Treatment Information
Gatto et al,[3] 2012	229	21 (9%)	3 (1%)	68 (30%)	Corticosteroids recommended
Fredi et al,[18] 2015	31	3 (9.6%)	6 (21%)	14 (45%)	Corticosteriods most common treatment, without evidence for improvement of outcomes
Iskender et al,[39] 2014	63	11 (17%)	6 (9.5%)	2 (3%)	Medications used during pregnancy: colchicine, corticosteroids, chloroquine

VASCULITIS TREATMENT IN PREGNANCY

The management of vasculitis during pregnancy is similar to the management of the disease outside of pregnancy, with only small modifications. Only 3 rheumatic medications are proven teratogens: methotrexate (MTX), mycophenolate (MMF), and cyclophosphamide (CYC).[40] Each of these teratogens doubles the risk for pregnancy loss. MTX doubles the risk for serious birth defects, although the overall risk is less than 10%.[41] First-trimester exposure to MMF or CYC places the fetus at about a 25% risk for any birth defect.[40,42] MTX, MMF, and CYC should be stopped before attempting conception; patients should be switched to lower-risk medications for pregnancy. If a pregnancy is conceived on these medications, the teratogen should be stopped immediately and the patient referred to obstetrics to discuss the risks of these drugs to the developing fetus.

The remaining medications most commonly used to manage vasculitis are considered relatively compatible with pregnancy. A general rule to follow is that the systemic inflammation of active vasculitis is typically more dangerous for a pregnancy, increasing the risks for pregnancy loss, fetal growth restriction, and preterm birth, than the nonteratogenic medications that are currently available. When stopping a teratogenic medication, it is strongly recommended to replace it with a low-risk alternative to minimize the risk of vasculitis flare.

Although rheumatologists seem to be most comfortable prescribing prednisone during pregnancy, this may not always be the best choice to manage disease during pregnancy, largely because of maternal effects. Prednisone has a myriad of possible risks in pregnancy, making it best reserved to acutely treat active inflammation. First-trimester exposure had been suggested to triple the risk for cleft lip and palate from 1 per 1000 in the general population to 3 per 1000 among pregnancies exposed to corticosteroids in a non–dose-dependent manner[43]; however, newer data suggest there is no increased risk.[44] Prednisone increases the risk for preterm birth and limits fetal growth significantly.[45] It also increases the risks for gestational diabetes, HTN, and excessive maternal weight gain, all manifestations that are associated with short- and long-term complications for the offspring and mother. Therefore, it is preferable to use nonteratogenic immunosuppressant medications to control vasculitis activity before and during pregnancy, holding prednisone in reserve for flares of disease during pregnancy.

The oral immunosuppressant azathioprine (AZA) has the greatest amount of data to support compatibility with pregnancy, followed by cyclosporine and tacrolimus.[40] These medications have been used for decades to treat women with solid organ transplants during pregnancy without an increase in birth defects or pregnancy loss. They can be started before conception and continued through pregnancy and into breastfeeding. There is some transplacental transfer of AZA, which may cause mild temporary immunosuppression in the offspring.

Tumor necrosis factor (TNF) inhibitors have been continued during pregnancy for women with inflammatory bowel disease (IBD) for the past decade.[46] Data on more than 1000 pregnancies have shown comparable pregnancy outcomes with women with IBD not on TNF inhibitors. MotherToBaby has been collecting prospective pregnancies with TNF-inhibitor exposure since Food and Drug Administration approval. Their study of etanercept suggests a 2-fold increase in serious birth defects but no pattern to these malformations, no increase in minor birth defects, and no increase in pregnancy losses.[47] Without a specific pattern of congenital anomalies, their association with underlying drug remains unconfirmed. The MotherToBaby study of adalimumab, on the other hand, found no increase in birth defects or other complications.[48] TNF inhibitors can be continued through the preconception period, pregnancy, and into lactation. The immunoglobulin G (IgG)–based TNF inhibitors cross the placenta starting around week 16, with increasing transfer closer to term. For this reason, these drugs should be held around gestational week 30 to 32 but can be restarted soon after delivery. Certolizumab does not have an Fc portion, limiting transfer across the placenta.[49] Infants with in utero TNF-inhibitor exposure should not be given live vaccines in the first 5 months of life: few live vaccines are given in this period, but live vaccines that may be considered during this period and should be held include *Rotavirus* and *bacillus Calmette-Guerin*. Exposed infants seem to respond normally to other vaccines and should be vaccinated on schedule to protect them from communicable diseases.[50]

Rituximab is an IgG antibody, so it crosses the placenta in the second half of pregnancy. Infusion in the latter part of pregnancy has been associated with an absence of B cells in the offspring, which can persist for months.[51] For this reason, rituximab is generally not infused later in pregnancy. It seems, however, that pregnancies conceived in the months following rituximab infusion are not at increased risk for complications. In addition, infusion early in pregnancy or in the months before conception may be an acceptable approach to the management of an ANCA-associated vasculitis that is flaring or that is at high risk for flaring without maintenance therapy.

Colchicine has been shown to be low risk in pregnancy in studies of women with BD and familial Mediterranean fever.[40] It has not been associated with birth defects, pregnancy loss, or preterm birth. Therefore, continuing colchicine throughout pregnancy may be a good way to manage BD and may allow these patients to avoid the use of prednisone.

SUMMARY

Although vasculitis is associated with increased pregnancy complications, tight control of disease activity during pregnancy can improve the chance for success. Stopping all medications for the specific purpose of pregnancy may increase the risk of flare of underlying disease, unless a woman has been known to remain in remission without medications. If not, then controlling disease with low-risk immunosuppressive medications and using prednisone briefly and in moderation yields the greatest chance for a healthy baby and mother.

REFERENCES

1. Doria A, Iaccarino L, Ghirardello A, et al. Pregnancy in rare autoimmune rheumatic diseases: UCTD, MCTD, myositis, systemic vasculitis and Behçet disease. Lupus 2004;13(9):690–5.
2. Doria A, Ghirardello A, Iaccarino L, et al. Pregnancy, cytokines, and disease activity in systemic lupus erythematosus. Arthritis Rheum 2004;51(6):989–95.
3. Gatto M, Iaccarino L, Canova M, et al. Pregnancy and vasculitis: a systematic review of the literature. Autoimmun Rev 2012;11(6–7):A447–59.
4. Zafar U, Sany O, Velmurugan U, et al. Wegener's granulomatosis in pregnancy: a multidisciplinary approach. J Obstet Gynaecol 2008;28(5):532–3.
5. Palit J, Clague RB. Wegener's granulomatosis presenting during first trimester of pregnancy. Br J Rheumatol 1990;29(5):389–90.
6. Koukoura O, Mantas N, Linardakis H, et al. Successful term pregnancy in a patient with Wegener's granulomatosis: case report and literature review. Fertil Steril 2008;89(2):457.e1-5.
7. Pagnoux C, Le Guern V, Goffinet F, et al. Pregnancies in systemic necrotizing vasculitides: report on 12 women and their 20 pregnancies. Rheumatology 2011;50(5):953–61.
8. Alfhaily F, Watts R, Leather A. Wegener's granulomatosis occurring de novo during pregnancy. Clin Exp Rheumatol 2009;27(1 Suppl 52):S86–8.
9. Cetinkaya R, Odabas AR, Gursan N, et al. Microscopic polyangiitis in a pregnant woman. South Med J 2002;95(12):1441–3.
10. Milne KL, Stanley KP, Temple RC, et al. Microscopic polyangiitis: first report of a case with onset during pregnancy. Nephrol Dial Transplant 2004;19(1):234–7.
11. Morton MR. Hypersensitivity vasculitis (microscopic polyangiitis) in pregnancy with transmission to the neonate. Br J Obstet Gynaecol 1998;105(8):928–30.
12. Debby A, Tanay A, Zakut H. Allergic granulomatosis and angiitis (Churg-Strauss vasculitis) in pregnancy. Int Arch Allergy Immunol 1993;102(3):307–8.

13. Pauzner R, Mayan H, Hershko E, et al. Exacerbation of Wegener's granulomatosis during pregnancy: report of a case with tracheal stenosis and literature review. J Rheumatol 1994;21(6):1153–6.
14. Parnham AP, Thatcher GN. Pregnancy and active Wegener granulomatosis. Aust N Z J Obstet Gynaecol 1996;36(3):361–3.
15. Connolly JO, Lanham JG, Partridge MR. Fulminant pregnancy-related Churg-Strauss syndrome. Br J Rheumatol 1994;33(8):776–7.
16. Abul-Haj SK, Flanagan P. Asthma associated with disseminated necrotizing granulomatous vasculitis, the Churg-Strauss syndrome. Report of a case. Med Ann Dist Columbia 1961;30:670–6.
17. Clowse ME, Richeson RL, Pieper C, et al. Pregnancy outcomes among patients with vasculitis. Arthritis Care Res 2013;65(8):1370–4.
18. Fredi M, Lazzaroni MG, Tani C, et al. Systemic vasculitis and pregnancy: a multicenter study on maternal and neonatal outcome of 65 prospectively followed pregnancies. Autoimmun Rev 2015;14(8):686–91.
19. Owen J, Hauth JC. Polyarteritis nodosa in pregnancy: a case report and brief literature review. Am J Obstet Gynecol 1989;160(3):606–7.
20. Pitkin RM. Polyarteritis nodosa. Clin Obstet Gynecol 1983;26(3):579–86.
21. Johnston SL, Lock RJ, Gompels MM. Takayasu arteritis: a review. J Clin Pathol 2002;55(7):481–6.
22. Jacquemyn Y, Vercauteren M. Pregnancy and Takayasu's arteritis of the pulmonary artery. J Obstet Gynaecol 2005;25(1):63–5.
23. Askie LM, Duley L, Henderson-Smart DJ, et al. Antiplatelet agents for prevention of pre-eclampsia: a meta-analysis of individual patient data. Lancet 2007; 369(9575):1791–8.
24. Sibai B, Dekker G, Kupferminc M. Pre-eclampsia. Lancet 2005;365(9461): 785–99.
25. Suri V, Aggarwal N, Keepanasseril A, et al. Pregnancy and Takayasu arteritis: a single centre experience from North India. J Obstet Gynaecol Res 2010;36(3): 519–24.
26. Ishikawa K, Matsuura S. Occlusive thromboaortopathy (Takayasu's disease) and pregnancy. Clinical course and management of 33 pregnancies and deliveries. Am J Cardiol 1982;50(6):1293–300.
27. Matsumura A, Moriwaki R, Numano F. Pregnancy in Takayasu arteritis from the view of internal medicine. Heart Vessels Suppl 1992;7:120–4.
28. Aso T, Abe S, Yaguchi T. Clinical gynecologic features of pregnancy in Takayasu arteritis. Heart Vessels Suppl 1992;7:125–32.
29. Sharma BK, Jain S, Vasishta K. Outcome of pregnancy in Takayasu arteritis. Int J Cardiol 2000;75(Suppl 1):S159–62.
30. Gasch O, Vidaller A, Pujol R. Takayasu arteritis and pregnancy from the point of view of the internist. J Rheumatol 2009;36(7):1554–5.
31. Umeda Y, Mori Y, Takagi H, et al. Abdominal aortic aneurysm related to Takayasu arteritis during pregnancy. Heart Vessels 2004;19(3):155–6.
32. Lakhi NA, Jones J. Takayasu's arteritis in pregnancy complicated by peripartum aortic dissection. Arch Gynecol Obstet 2010;282(1):103–6.
33. Assad AP, da Silva TF, Bonfa E, et al. Maternal and neonatal outcomes in 89 patients with Takayasu arteritis (TA): comparison before and after the TA diagnosis. J Rheumatol 2015;42(10):1861–4.
34. Comarmond C, Mirault T, Biard L, et al. Takayasu arteritis and pregnancy. Arthritis Rheumatol 2015;67(12):3262–9.

35. Wechsler B, Genereau T, Biousse V, et al. Pregnancy complicated by cerebral venous thrombosis in Behcet's disease. Am J Obstet Gynecol 1995;173(5): 1627–9.
36. Jadaon J, Shushan A, Ezra Y, et al. Behcet's disease and pregnancy. Acta Obstet Gynecol Scand 2005;84(10):939–44.
37. el Hajoui S, Nabil S, Khachani M, et al. Pregnancy in patients with Behcet's disease. Presse Med 2002;31(1 Pt 1):19–20 [in French].
38. Komaba H, Takeda Y, Fukagawa M. Extensive deep vein thrombosis in a postpartum woman with Behcet's disease associated with nephrotic syndrome. Kidney Int 2007;71(1):6.
39. Iskender C, Yasar O, Kaymak O, et al. Behcet's disease and pregnancy: a retrospective analysis of course of disease and pregnancy outcome. J Obstet Gynaecol Res 2014;40(6):1598–602.
40. Gotestam Skorpen C, Hoeltzenbein M, Tincani A, et al. The EULAR points to consider for use of antirheumatic drugs before pregnancy, and during pregnancy and lactation. Ann Rheum Dis 2016;75(5):795–810.
41. Weber-Schoendorfer C, Chambers C, Wacker E, et al. Pregnancy outcome after methotrexate treatment for rheumatic disease prior to or during early pregnancy: a prospective multicenter cohort study. Arthritis Rheumatol 2014;66(5):1101–10.
42. Sifontis NM, Coscia LA, Constantinescu S, et al. Pregnancy outcomes in solid organ transplant recipients with exposure to mycophenolate mofetil or sirolimus. Transplantation 2006;82(12):1698–702.
43. Park-Wyllie L, Mazzotta P, Pastuszak A, et al. Birth defects after maternal exposure to corticosteroids: prospective cohort study and meta-analysis of epidemiological studies. Teratology 2000;62(6):385–92.
44. Bay Bjorn AM, Ehrenstein V, Hundborg HH, et al. Use of corticosteroids in early pregnancy is not associated with risk of oral clefts and other congenital malformations in offspring. Am J Ther 2014;21(2):73–80.
45. Clark CA, Spitzer KA, Nadler JN, et al. Preterm deliveries in women with systemic lupus erythematosus. J Rheumatol 2003;30(10):2127–32.
46. Nguyen GC, Seow CH, Maxwell C, et al. The Toronto consensus statements for the management of inflammatory bowel disease in pregnancy. Gastroenterology 2016;150(3):734–57.e1.
47. Chambers CD, Johnson DL, Luo Y, et al. Pregnancy outcome in women treated with etanercept: an update on the OTIS Autoimmune Diseases in Pregnancy Project. The Teratology Scociety Annual Meeting. Montreal (Canada), July, 2015.
48. Chambers C, Johnson D, Luo Y, et al. Pregnancy outcome in women treated with adalimumab for rheumatoid arthritis: an update on the OTIS autoimmune diseases in pregnancy project. Paper presented at: 31st International Conference on Pharmacoepidemiology & Therapeutic Risk Management 2015. Boston, August, 2015.
49. Mahadevan U, Wolf DC, Dubinsky M, et al. Placental transfer of anti-tumor necrosis factor agents in pregnant patients with inflammatory bowel disease. Clin Gastroenterol Hepatol 2013;11(3):286–92 [quiz: e224].
50. Sheibani S, Cohen R, Kane S, et al. The effect of maternal peripartum anti-TNFalpha use on infant immune response. Dig Dis Sci 2016;61(6):1622–7.
51. Chakravarty EF, Murray ER, Kelman A, et al. Pregnancy outcomes after maternal exposure to rituximab. Blood 2011;117(5):1499–506.

Lactation and Management of Postpartum Disease

Bonnie L. Bermas, MD

KEYWORDS

- Rheumatologic diseases • Postpartum flare • DMARDs • Biologics • Lactation

KEY POINTS

- Rheumatologic diseases, such as rheumatoid arthritis (RA) and systemic lupus erythematosus (SLE), may flare in the postpartum period.
- There are many benefits of breastfeeding to both the mother and the infant; fortunately, many but not all medications used to manage rheumatic diseases can be continued in breastfeeding women.
- Short-acting nonsteroidal anti-inflammatory drugs (NSAIDs), low-dose aspirin, glucocorticoids in doses under 20 mg a day, antimalarials, azathioprine, tacrolimus, cyclosporine, most tumor necrosis factor (TNF)-α blockers, anakinra, and intravenous immunoglobulin (IVIG) are compatible with nursing.
- Methotrexate and cyclophosphamide are not considered compatible with nursing.
- Insufficient data on the safety of leflunomide, mycophenolate mofetil, tofacitinib, rituximab, belimumab, abatacept, tocilizumab, golimumab, and secukinumab in lactation exist.

Rheumatic diseases have a preferential impact on women. Therefore, issues concerning family planning are important considerations for rheumatologists. There is limited information regarding the postpartum period and lactation in rheumatic disease patients; nonetheless, evidence suggests that many rheumatologic disorders flare after delivery. This risk of disease activity coupled with limitations in medication use during breastfeeding make the postpartum period particularly challenging for women with rheumatologic diseases. This article discusses disease activity during the postpartum period and reviews the safety during lactation of commonly used medications for the management of rheumatic diseases.

IMMUNE SYSTEM DURING PREGNANCY AND THE POSTPARTUM PERIOD

The immune system changes throughout pregnancy and the postpartum period. During early pregnancy, a proinflammatory state exists to facilitate implantation. Type 1 helper T cells producing interleukin (IL)-6, IL-8, and TNF-α predominate, and natural killer cells contribute to local inflammation by producing chemokines and

Division of Rheumatology, Immunology and Allergy, Brigham and Women's Hospital, BTM 60 Fenwood Road, Boston, MA 02115, USA
E-mail address: bbermas@partners.org

Rheum Dis Clin N Am 43 (2017) 249–262
http://dx.doi.org/10.1016/j.rdc.2016.12.002
0889-857X/17/© 2017 Elsevier Inc. All rights reserved.

rheumatic.theclinics.com

angiogenic factors.[1] After implantation, however, levels of IL-8 and IL-1β decrease until rising in the postpartum period.[2] The second trimester becomes a relatively anti-inflammatory state to facilitate fetal growth and development. Toward the end of pregnancy, the immunologic milieu becomes proinflammatory again to promote labor and delivery.[3] For this reason, infections that trigger proinflammatory cytokines can increase the risk of preterm delivery.[4] These immunologic changes toward the end of pregnancy are thought to have an impact on disease activity during the postpartum period.

DISEASE ACTIVITY DURING PREGNANCY AND THE POSTPARTUM PERIOD

Historically, RA is reported to improve during pregnancy in approximately 75% of patients.[5] More recent data suggest that this number is closer to 50%.[6] In contrast, the data on SLE are variable.[7] SLE patients who have stable disease for the 6 months preceding pregnancy and no history of renal disease tend to do well, whereas primigravidas, women with prior renal disease or recently active disease, and those who discontinue hydroxychloroquine tend to flare during pregnancy.[8–10]

The postpartum period is challenging for all women but particularly for those with rheumatic diseases: flares can cause fatigue, myalgias, and joint pain that may make caring for a newborn difficult. In 1 study of 140 women with inflammatory arthritis, 66% reported worsening symptoms in the first 6 months postpartum.[11] In another prospective study, 50% of RA women had increased disease activity after delivery.[6] Women with SLE also have an increased risk of flare postpartum.[12,13] One study found 35% of SLE patients flared in the first 8 weeks postpartum, a significantly higher rate than in the nonpregnant control group.[12]

LACTATION

Lactation is associated with a complex feedback system involving the pituitary that includes release of prolactin to stimulate milk production. Prolactin also increases TNF-α expression in peripheral CD14 monocytes of RA patients[14] and, clinically, breastfeeding has been associated with postpartum flare in RA.[15] In contrast, epidemiologic studies suggest that breastfeeding reduces the risk of new onset of RA.[16] In patients with SLE, elevated levels of prolactin may increase flares.[17] Bromocriptine, which blocks prolactin release, has been used to treat both SLE and RA. A randomized controlled study of 76 women with SLE followed in the postpartum period compared patients who received a 14-day course of bromocriptine (2.5 mg twice a day) to those who did not: 6 months to 12 months after delivery, Systemic Lupus Erythematosus Disease Activity Index (SLEDAI) scores as well as steroid and immunosuppressive medication use were significantly lower in the bromocriptine-treated group.[18] Although similar benefits have been reported in RA,[19] a recent placebo-controlled trial of 88 RA women treated with bromocriptine failed to show improvement.[20]

BREASTFEEDING

The benefits of human milk during early infancy include better nutrition, improved gastrointestinal function, and enhanced immunity to pathogens[21–23]; long-term benefits include reduced risk of obesity, cancer, heart disease, and diabetes.[24–26] For the mother, breastfeeding may reduce stress, improve mother-infant bonding,[27] enhance postpartum weight loss,[28] and, long-term, reduce cardiovascular risk.[29] The American Academy of Pediatrics (AAP) and the American Association of Family Practitioners recommend exclusive breastfeeding for the first 6 months and continued breastfeeding for an additional 6 months.[30,31] Despite the clear benefits, however, in 2013 only 51.8% of infants were breastfed: 44.4% of infants were breastfed exclusively through 3 months and 22.3% exclusively through 6 months.[32] Although specific data on rates of breastfeeding among women with rheumatic diseases are limited, 1 study of breastfeeding in SLE mothers found that 49% of women breastfed,[33] a figure similar to that reported in the general population.

BREAST MILK

During the second half of pregnancy, lactogenesis, or the secretion of breast milk, begins. Small amounts are secreted beginning at 16 weeks' gestation[34] and large amounts are produced after delivery. Breast milk is composed of lactose and oligosaccharides, milk fat, proteins including immunoglobulin (Ig) A, and minerals. Synthesis and secretion occur by 5 mechanisms: exocytosis for proteins and lactose, reversed pinocytosis for fat, transcytosis for intact proteins, apical transport for electrolytes, and paracellular movement. Maternal medications are transferred by diffusion of unbound drug.[35,36] Lipid-soluble, low-molecular-weight, nonionized and non–protein-bound medications cross most easily into breast milk; in addition, drugs with longer half-lives accumulate in higher concentrations.

MEDICATIONS DURING LACTATION

Milk-to-plasma ratios are used to evaluate drug safety during lactation: safe levels are defined as breast milk levels of less than 10% the infant therapeutic dose or the maternal weight-adjusted dose in milligrams/kilogram. The total volume of ingested milk also influences drug exposure. Peak levels of drug occur 1 to 2 hours after ingestion; however, milk level and infant serum level are not the same, because absorption through the infant gastrointestinal tract also has an impact on serum level. For example, IgG is largely degraded by infant gastrointestinal tract enzymes so is not absorbed in significant amounts. Gestational age at birth also has an impact on infant serum level: premature infants have more difficulty metabolizing medications, leading to higher drug concentration, and those who have a poorly developed gastrointestinal tract may absorb more than full-term infants.

Determining drug safety during lactation is challenging: conclusions are often based on case reports or a lack of reassuring information. For example, the recommendation that methotrexate be avoided by lactating women by the British Society for Rheumatology/British Health Professionals in Rheumatology (BSR/BHPR) is based on insufficient information regarding safety rather than adverse findings.[37,38] Proceedings from an American College of Rheumatology Reproductive Health Summit identified the exclusion of breastfeeding women from clinical trials and inadequate information regarding drug metabolism and transfer to breast milk as 2 important factors that contribute to knowledge gaps in drug safety in lactation.[39] Similarly, the Food and Drug Administration recognized that the existing labeling for safety of medications in pregnancy and lactation was not sufficient and revamped their labeling.[40] Safety during lactation of commonly used medications for management of rheumatic diseases is reviewed later (**Tables 1** and **2**).

NONSTEROIDAL ANTI-INFLAMMATORY DRUGS AND ASPIRIN

Nonselective NSAIDs are weak acids that are highly protein bound; as a result, little drug is excreted in breast milk. In general, shorter-acting medications, such as ibuprofen, are preferable because they are less likely to accumulate in breast milk at

Table 1
Summary of current lactation data on antirheumatic drugs

Medication	Breast Milk Levels	Infant Serum Levels	Safety in Lactation	Comments
NSAIDs	Low	Low	Compatible	NSAIDs with shorter half-life preferable
Low-dose aspirin	Low	Low	Compatible	Avoid doses greater than 100 mg/d
Prednisone, prednisolone	Low	Low	Compatible	In doses greater than 20–50 mg/d, avoid breastfeeding for 4 h after dose
Hydroxychloroquine, chloroquine	Low	No data	Compatible	Long-term follow-up of infants: no evidence of retinal disease
Sulfasalazine	Moderate	Variable	Compatible	Bloody diarrhea in infant reported; avoid in premature infants
Azathioprine	Low	No drug	Compatible	
Cyclosporine	Variable	Variable	Compatible	Consider infant serum creatinine and drug levels
Tacrolimus	Low	Low	Compatible	
Mycophenolate mofetil	No data	No data	Unknown	Avoid
Methotrexate	Low	No data	Potential risk-avoid	
Cyclophosphamide	Passes into breast milk	No data	High risk	Hypothetical risk of immune suppression and carcinogenesis
Leflunomide	No data	No data	Likely high risk	
Etanercept	Low	Low	Compatible	
Adalimumab	Low	No data	Compatible	
Infliximab	Low	No data	Compatible	
Certolizumab pegol	Low	No data	Compatible	
Anakinra	No data	No data	Compatible	
IVIG	Transfers	No data	Compatible	
Abatacept	No data	No data		High molecular weight makes transfer into breast milk unlikely
Tocilizumab	No data	No data		High molecular weight makes transfer into breast milk unlikely
Rituximab	No data	No data		High molecular weight makes transfer into breast milk unlikely
Belimumab	No data	No data		High molecular weight makes transfer into breast milk unlikely

(continued on next page)

Table 1
(continued)

Medication	Breast Milk Levels	Infant Serum Levels	Safety in Lactation	Comments
Golimumab	No data	No data		High molecular weight makes transfer into breast milk unlikely
Secukinumab	No data	No data		High molecular weight makes transfer into breast milk unlikely
Tofacitinib	No data	No data	Avoid	Low molecular weight makes transfer into breast milk likely

significant concentrations. In 1 study of 12 patients taking 400 mg of ibuprofen every 6 hours, no ibuprofen was detectable in the breast milk.[41] In another report, a woman taking 2400 mg of ibuprofen over a 42-hour interval had 10 breast milk samples collected: the calculated dose for the infant was less than 0.0008% of the mother's dose.[42] The AAP concludes that ibuprofen is compatible with breastfeeding.[43] Some investigators suggest that due to antiplatelet effects, nonselective NSAIDs should be avoided in women nursing neonates with thrombocytopenia.[44] Piroxicam, a longer-acting NSAID, has a higher concentration in breast milk, but the average weight-adjusted infant dose is only 3.5% of the maternal dose,[45] well within safe levels.

Aspirin is secreted into breast milk in low concentration[46]; however, there has been a report of infant toxicity from salicylates in a breastfeeding infant whose mother was taking 650 mg of aspirin every 4 hours.[47] The BSR/BHPR suggest that although low-dose aspirin is probably safe, high-dose aspirin should be avoided.[38]

Celecoxib is a cyclooxygenase (COX)-2 inhibitor. In 1 breastfeeding mother taking 100 mg of celecoxib twice daily, the maximum calculated infant dose was 40 µg/kg daily.[48]

Table 2
Summary of current lactation data on other drugs commonly used in rheumatology practice

Medication	Breast Milk Level	Infant Sera Level	Safety	Comments
ACE inhibitors (enalapril and captopril)	Minimal	Unknown	Compatible	
ARBs	No data	No data	Unknown	
Nifedipine	Minimal	No data	Compatible	Can be used to manage nipple Raynaud syndrome
Anticoagulants				
Warfarin	Undetected	Unknown	Compatible	
Heparin	No data	No data	Unknown	
Low-molecular-weight heparin	No data	No data	Compatible	Large molecule, probably safe
Colchicine	Transferred to breast milk	No data	Compatible	

In another 6 lactating mothers taking celecoxib, 200 mg a day, the estimated dose for infants was 13 μg/kg.[49] These data suggest that celecoxib is compatible with nursing.

GLUCOCORTICOIDS

Little prednisone is transferred into human breast milk.[50] In 1 series of 124 transplant recipients who nursed while taking low doses of prednisone, none of the infants had health issues.[51] A report of 6 women given 10 mg to 80 mg of prednisolone daily found that minimal amounts of prednisolone were transferred to breast milk at doses under 20 mg and that at the highest dose, less than 0.1% the maternal dose would be ingested by the nursing infant. The investigators recommended waiting 4 hours after doses greater than 20 mg of prednisolone to nurse.[52] A recent recommendation from the European League Against Rheumatism (EULAR) is more liberal, suggesting a 4-hour delay only if taking greater than or equal to 50 mg prednisone daily.[53] Prednisone and prednisolone are compatible with breastfeeding; at higher doses, mothers should consider waiting 4 hours after medication to resume nursing.

ANTIMALARIALS

The antimalarials hydroxychloroquine and chloroquine are the mainstay of therapy for SLE. Antimalarials are weak bases with a long half-life, and minimal drug is transferred to breast milk.[54,55] In breast milk samples from a woman taking hydroxychloroquine, 200 mg twice daily, mean drug concentration was 1.1 mg/L; the calculated daily infant dose was 1.1 mg, or 2% of the maternal dose on a body-weight basis.[56] Estimates of infant sera concentrations of chloroquine in exclusively breastfed infants range from .55% to 2.3% of the maternal weight-adjusted dose.[57,58] Infants of mothers treated through pregnancy and lactation with hydroxychloroquine have not shown any retinal, motor, or growth abnormalities.[59] The AAP considers hydroxychloroquine and chloroquine compatible with nursing.[43]

SULFASALAZINE

Sulfasalazine is secreted at low concentrations into breast milk; however, the metabolite sulfapyridine is transferred at levels 30% to 60% of maternal serum.[60–62] There has been 1 report of bloody diarrhea in a 2-month-old breastfed infant whose mother was taking 3 g/d of sulfasalazine, which resolved after discontinuation.[63] For this reason, the AAP advises caution in prescribing sulfasalazine to lactating women[30]; other professional organizations suggest limiting breastfeeding to full-term infants.[37,38,52]

IMMUNOSUPPRESSIVE DRUGS

The immunosuppressive agents azathioprine, cyclosporine, mycophenolate mofetil, and tacrolimus have long been used to prevent graft rejection in transplant recipients and are now commonly used in management of rheumatologic diseases. Azathioprine is metabolized to 6-mercaptopurine, and it is this metabolite that appears in breast milk at reported levels of 0.07% to 1% of the maternal weight-adjusted dosage.[64–66] The impact of azathioprine on clinical parameters in breastfed infants is likewise reassuring: in 1 study of 30 infants of mothers who took azathioprine during pregnancy and lactation, 20 infants had white blood cell counts performed: only 1 infant had a low white blood cell count that subsequently resolved.[67] The AAP, BSR/BHPR, and recent EULAR recommendations suggest that azathioprine is compatible with nursing.[37,43,53]

Reports on cyclosporine levels in breast milk are more variable. In 1 study of 7 mothers, breast milk levels ranged from 50 µg to 227 µg/L and the calculated infant dose of cyclosporine was less than 300 µg daily, well below 10% of the maternal dose.[68] In contrast, however, in a study of 5 mother-infant pairs, 1 infant had levels of cyclosporine approximately 78% of the weight-normalized maternal dose, essentially a therapeutic infant dose.[69] This infant had normal growth and development at 18 months; however, this finding suggests that breastfed infants of mothers taking cyclosporine should be monitored for drug levels and renal function. The AAP suggests this medication may interfere with cellular metabolism of nursing infants[30] and recommends avoiding cyclosporine in lactating women; however, the recent EULAR and BSR/BHPR recommendations suggest compatibility with nursing.[37,53]

Tacrolimus has assumed a growing role in management of lupus nephritis and available data suggest that little drug is transferred to breast milk. In breast milk samples from 6 mothers taking tacrolimus, drug concentrations averaged 0.79 ng/mL and the calculated average infant dose was less than 0.1 µg/kg/d, well below the dose used to prevent pediatric rejection.[70] In another study of 6 treated women who breastfed, 4 infants had tacrolimus levels that were undetectable.[71] The AAP, EULAR, and BSR/BHPR consider tacrolimus compatible with nursing.[37,43,52]

METHOTREXATE

Methotrexate, a folic acid antagonist, is the cornerstone of therapy for RA and other inflammatory conditions. In 1 lactating woman who received 22.5 mg of methotrexate daily for choriocarcinoma, levels in the breast milk during the first 3 days after administration ranged from 2.3 µg/L to 2.7 µg/L. The estimated cumulative dose excreted in the milk during the first 12 hours was 0.32 µg, well under 10% of the maternal mg/kg dose.[72] In another woman who received a 25-mg subcutaneous dose of methotrexate for RA, milk levels averaged 22.7 µg/L. The investigators calculated that a fully breastfed infant would receive 1% of weight-adjusted maternal dosing.[73] Despite these reassuring data, most professional societies caution against breastfeeding in women who are taking methotrexate.[37,43,53]

CYCLOPHOSPHAMIDE

Although cyclophosphamide appears in breast milk of treated women, an exact amount has not been quantified.[74] There are 2 reports of leukopenia, however, in infants exposed to cyclophosphamide during breastfeeding.[75,76] Recommendations from professional organizations are to avoid breastfeeding.[37,43,53]

BIOLOGICS

Biologic therapies have transformed management of SLE, RA, and vasculitis. TNF-α inhibitors and other biologics are unlikely to be transferred to human breast milk in significant concentration due to their large molecular weight and given that little IgG1 is secreted into breast milk. Moreover, these drugs are likely to be enzymatically degraded by the infant gastrointestinal system.

TUMOR NECROSIS FACTOR-α INHIBITORS

Etanercept is transferred to breast milk in low concentration; case reports suggest breast milk levels ranging from 3.5 µg/L to 7.5 µg/L.[77–79] One exclusively breastfed infant, whose mother received etanercept throughout pregnancy and postpartum, was noted to have a serum etanercept levels of 21 µg/L at 1 week of age but an undetectable level at 12 weeks.[77] Peak levels of adalimumab in breast milk (31 μg/L) occur 6 days after injection of a 40-mg dose,[80] with undetectable drug levels in breastfed infants' sera.[81,82] Minimal to no levels of infliximab have been detected in breast milk of treated nursing mothers.[83–85] One report of a breastfed infant exposed to infliximab in utero up to 2 weeks prior to delivery revealed an infant serum level of 39.5 μg/L/mg. Despite continued maternal therapy and resumption of breastfeeding at 10 weeks, the infant's infliximab level continued to drop,[83] suggesting the majority of drug transfer was due to placental transfer and not lactation. Certolizumab is also considered compatible with nursing: case reports of 6 women treated while nursing failed to show detectable drug in breast milk.[86] There are no human data on the safety of breastfeeding in mothers treated with golimumab, although a study showed no adverse effects on breastfed infant macaques.[87] These data as a whole suggest that TNF-α inhibitors are compatible with nursing, a suggestion supported by several professional organizations.[37,53]

TOCILIZUMAB

Data are limited for tocilizumab, although there is 1 report of 2 women who resumed tocilizumab postpartum and breastfed their infants. Although breast milk and infant sera levels were not reported, there were no untoward effects reported.[88]

ANAKINRA

Anakinra is a human IL-1 receptor antagonist (IL-1Ra). IL-1Ra is a normal component of breast milk.[89] Although there are no data on the transfer of anakinra to breast milk, there is a case report of 1 woman with adult-onset Still disease receiving anakinra, 100 mg daily, throughout pregnancy and lactation whose infant had normal growth and development.[90] EULAR consensus was that this medication may be continued during breastfeeding.[53]

INTRAVENOUS IMMUNOGLOBULIN

Reported data on IVIG and breastfeeding are limited. In 2 mothers who received IVIG while lactating, 1 had normal levels and the other had elevated levels of IVIG in the breast milk.[91] In a series of 69 women who received IVIG postpartum, none of their breastfed infants had adverse effects.[92] IVIG is considered compatible with breastfeeding.[53]

MEDICATIONS WITH UNKNOWN RISK

There are currently no data on the safety of mycophenolate mofetil or leflunomide, and recommendations are to avoid these medications in lactating women.[37] Although there are no data on safety of nursing while on the biologics rituximab, belimumab, abatacept or secukinumab, the large size of these molecules makes significant breast milk transfer unlikely. In contrast, tofacitinib's small size suggests it readily enters breast milk and should be avoided in lactating women.

OTHER MEDICATIONS
Antihypertensives

Angiotensin-converting enzyme (ACE) inhibitors and angiotensin II receptor blockers (ARBs) are important for management of hypertension associated with many rheumatic diseases. Although information is not available on all of the ACE inhibitors, data on enalapril and captopril suggest minimal to no transfer to breast milk.[93–95] There is no information on infant serum levels; however, no adverse effects have been reported in breastfed infants exposed to ACE inhibitors. A potential concern regarding ACE inhibitors is the hypothetical reduction in serum prolactin reported in hypertensive men.[96] Given that the prolactin level in lactating women is so much higher than in nonlactating men, however, it seems unlikely that these medications would have an impact on milk production. Nonetheless, there has been 1 report of a woman unable to produce adequate breast milk while taking captopril, 300 mg a day.[97] There are no available data on the compatibility of ARBs with breastfeeding.

Raynaud syndrome is common in women with rheumatic disorders; Raynaud syndrome affecting the nipple is rare but when it occurs it can impede nursing.[97] Calcium channel blockers are effective treatments. One study of women taking up to 30 mg nifedipine daily calculated the infant dose would be 8 μg/kg/d, less than 1.8% of the therapeutic pediatric dose,[98] suggesting compatibility with nursing.

Anticoagulants

Warfarin is considered compatible with nursing: studies have not identified detectable levels of drug in breast milk of treated mothers.[99] In another report, a breastfed infant of a warfarin-treated mother had a normal international normalized ratio (INR) despite the mother's supratherapeutic INR of 10.[100]

There are no data regarding the transference of heparin to breast milk; however, given its large size, it is unlikely to be transferred in significant amounts. Twelve infants breastfed by mothers receiving enoxaparin had normal serum factor Xa levels, suggesting that little of the drug is transferred to breast milk.[101]

Colchicine

Although colchicine is excreted in breast milk at levels that approach 10% of maternal serum levels,[102] a report of 10 infants of colchicine-treated mothers found no adverse effects on the infants.[103] The AAP considers colchicine compatible with breastfeeding.

SUMMARY

The postpartum period presents challenges to clinicians caring for rheumatic disease patients because it is not uncommon for these disorders to flare. Management is complicated because not all rheumatology medications are compatible with nursing. Given the benefits of breastfeeding for both mother and infant, all efforts should be made to choose medications compatible with lactation when possible (see **Tables 1** and **2**). There is a fine balance between maintaining optimal disease control and encouraging breastfeeding in women with rheumatic diseases. Communication regarding the most currently available data on medications is critical: maternal risk from poorly controlled disease must be weighed against the at times unknown effects on a nursing infant. This allows both providers and patients to make informed decisions during a joyful but unpredictable period.

REFERENCES

1. Mor G, Cardenas I, Abrahams V, et al. Inflammation and pregnancy: the role of the immune system at the implantation site. Ann NY Acad Sci 2011; 1221:80–7.
2. Christian LM, Porter K. Longitudinal changes in serum proinflammatory markers across pregnancy and post partum: effects of maternal body mass index. Cyokine 2014;70:134–40.

3. Mor G, Cardenas I. Review article: the immune system in pregnancy: a unique complexity. Am J Reprod Immunol 2010;63:425–33.
4. Romero R, Espinoza J, Goncalves LF, et al. Inflammation in preterm and term labour and delivery. Semin Fetal Neonatal Med 2006;11:317–26.
5. Nelson JL, Ostensen M. Pregnancy and rheumatoid arthritis. Rheum Dis Clin North Am 1997;23:195–212.
6. de Man YA, Dolhain RJ, van de Geijn FE, et al. Disease activity of rheumatoid arthritis during pregnancy: results from a nationwide prospective study. Arthritis Rheum 2008;59:1241–8.
7. Lockshin MD. Does Lupus Flare during pregnancy? Lupus 1993;2:1–2.
8. Borella E, Lojacono A, Gatto M, et al. Predictors of maternal and fetal complications in SLE patients: a prospective study. Immunol Res 2014;60:170–6.
9. Clowse ME, Magder L, Witter F, et al. Hydroxychlorquine in lupus pregnancy. Arthritis Rheum 2006;54:3640–7.
10. Saavedra MA, Sanchez A, Morales S, et al. Primigravida is associated with flare in women with systemic lupus erythematosus. Lupus 2016;24:180–5.
11. Barrett JH, Brennan P, Fiddler M, et al. Does rheumatoid arthritis remit during pregnancy and relapse postpartum? Results from a nationwide study in the United Kingdom performed prospectively from late pregnancy. Arthritis Rheum 1999;42:1219–27.
12. Ruiz-Irastorza G, Lima F, Alvez J, et al. Increased rate of lupus flare during pregnancy and the puerperium:a prospective study of 78 pregnancies. Br J Rheumatol 1996;35:133–8.
13. Liu J, Zhao Y, Song Y, et al. Pregnancy in women with systemic lupus erythematosus: a retrospective study of 111 pregnancies in Chinese women. J Matern Fetal Neonatal Med 2012;25:261–6.
14. Tang C, Li Y, Lin X, et al. Prolactin increases tumor necrosis factor alpha expression in peripheral CD14 monocytes of patients with rheumatoid arthritis. Cell Immunol 2014;290:164–8.
15. Barrett JH, Brennan P, Fiddler M, et al. Breast-feeding and postpartum relapse in women with rheumatoid and inflammatory arthritis. Arthritis Rheum 2000;43:1010–5.
16. Karlson EW, Mandl LA, Hankinson SE, et al. Do breast-feeding and other reproductive factors influence future risk of rheumatoid arthritis? Results from the Nurses Health Study. Arthritis Rheum 2004;50:3458–67.
17. Walker SE, Mcmurray RW, Houri JM, et al. Effects of prolactin in stimulating disease activity in systemic lupus erythematosus. Ann NY Acad Sci 1998;840:762–72.
18. Qian Q, Liuquin L, Hao L, et al. The effects of bromocriptine on preventing postpartum flare in systemic lupus erythematosuspatients from South China. J Immunol Res 2015;2015:316965.
19. McMurray RW. Bromocriptine in rheumatic and autoimmune diseases. Semin Arthritis Rheum 2001;31:21–32.
20. Salesi M, Sadeghihaddadzavareh S, Nasri P, et al. The role of bromocriptine int he treatment of patients with active rheumatoid arthritis. Int J Rheum Dis 2013;16:662–6.
21. Sheard NF, Walker WA. The role of breast milk in the development of the gastrointestinal tract. Nutr Rev 1988;46:1–8.
22. Hanson LA, Ahlstedt S, Andersson B, et al. Protective factors in milk and the development of the immune system. Pediatrics 1985;75:172–6.

23. Ladomenou F, Moschandreas J, Kafatos A, et al. Protective effect of exclusive breastfeeding against infections during infancy: a prospective study. Arch Dis Child 2010;95:1004–8.
24. Armstrong J, Reilly JJ. Breastfeeding and lowering the risk of childhood obesity. Lancet 2003;2002:359.
25. Davis MK, Savitz DA, Graubard BI. Infant feeding and childhood cancer. Lancet 1988;2:365–8.
26. Horta BL, Loret de Mola C, Victora CG. Long-term consequences of breastfeeding on cholesterol, obesity, systolic blood pressure and type 2 diabetes: a systemic review and meta –analysis. Acta Paediatr 2015;104:30.
27. Carter CS, Alternus M. Integrative functions of lactational hormones in social behavior and stress management. Ann NY Acad Sci 1997;807:164–74.
28. Dewey KG, Heinig MJ, Nommsen LA. Maternal weight-loss patterns during prolonged lactation. Am J Clin Nutr 1993;58:162–6.
29. Schwarz EB, Ray RM, Stuebe AM, et al. Duration of lactation and risk factors for maternal cardiovascular disease. Obstet Gynecol 2009;113:974–82.
30. American Academy of Pediatrics. Breastfeeding and the use of human milk. Pediatrics 2012;129:600–3.
31. Hauk L. AAFP releases position paper on breastfeeding. Am Fam Physician 2015;91:56–7.
32. National Immunization Survey Breastfeeding CDC 2002-2013, 2013 data. Available at: https://www.cdc.gov/breastfeeding/data/NIS_data/.
33. Noviani M, Wasserman S, Clowse MEB. Breastfeeding in mothers with systemic lupus erythematosus. Lupus 2016;25:973–9.
34. Neveille MC, Morton J, Umemura S. Lactogenesis. The transition from pregnancy to lactation. Pediatr Clin North Am 2001;48:35–52.
35. Neville MC. Anatomy and physiology of lactation. Pediatr Clin North Am 2001; 48:13–34.
36. Newton ER. Lactation and breastfeeding. In: Gabbe SG, Nielby JR, Simpson JL, et al, editors. Obstetrics: normal and problem pregnancies. 7th edition. Philadelphia: Sanders (Elsevier); 2017. p. 517–48.
37. Flint J, Panchal S, Hurrell A, et al. BSR and BHPR guideline on prescribing drugs in pregnancy and breastfeeding—Part I: standard and biologic disease modifying anti-rheumatic drugs and corticosteroids. Rheumatology (Oxford) 2016;55(9):1693–7.
38. Flint J, Panchal S, Hurrell A, et al. BSR and BHPR guideline on prescribing drugs in pregnancy and breastfeeding—Part II: analgesics and other drugs used in rheumatology practice. Rheumatology 2016;55(9):1698–702.
39. Kavanaugh A, Cush JJ, Ahmed MS, et al. Proceedings from the American College of Rheumatology Reproductive Health Summit: the management of fertility, pregnancy, and lactation in women with autoimmune and systemic inflammatory diseases. Arthritis Care Res (Hoboken) 2015;67:313–25.
40. Food and Drug Administration HHS. Content and format of labeling for human presctiption drug and biological products; requirements for pregnancy and lactation labeling. Final Rule. Fed Regist 2014;79:2063–103.
41. Townsend RJ, Benedetti TJ, Erickson SH, et al. Excretion of ibuprofen into breast milk. Am J Obstet Gynecol 1984;149:184–6.
42. Walter K, Dilger C. Ibuprofen in human milk. Br J Clin Pharmacol 1997;44:211–2.
43. American Academy of Pediatrics Committee on Drugs. The transfer of drugs and other chemicals into human milk. Pediatrics 2001;108:776–89.

44. Bloor M, Paech M. Nonsteroidal anti-inflammatory drugs during pregnancy and the initiation of lactation. Anesth Analg 2013;116:1063–75.
45. Ostensen M, Matheson I, Laufen H. Piroxicam in breast milk after long-term treatment. Eur J Clin Pharmacol 1988;35:567–9.
46. Bailey DN, Welbert RT, Naylor A. A study of salicylate and caffeine excretion in the breast milk of two nursing mothers. J Anal Toxicol 1982;6:64–8.
47. Clark JH, Wilson WG. A 16-day-old breast-fed infant with metabolic acidosis caused by salicylate. Clin Pediatr 1981;20:53–4.
48. Knoppert DC, Stempak D, Baruchel S, et al. Celecoxib in human milk: a case report. Pharmacotherapy 2003;23:97–100.
49. Ruhlen RL, Chen YC, Rottinghaus GE, et al. RE:"Transfer of celecoxib into human milk". J Hum Lact 2007;23:13–4.
50. Katz FH, Duncan BR. Entry of prednisone into human milk [letter]. N Engl J Med 1975;293:1154.
51. Constantinescu S, Pai A, Coscia LA, et al. Breast-feeding after transplantation. Best Pract Res Clin Obstet Gynaecol 2014;28:1163–73.
52. Ost L, Wettrell G, Bjorkhem I, et al. Prednisolone excretion in human milk. J Pediatr 1985;106:1008–11.
53. Gotestam Skorpen C, Hoeltzenbein M, Tincani A, et al. The EULAR points to consider for use of antirheumatic drugs before pregnancy, and during pregnancy and lactation. Ann Rheum Dis 2016;75:795–810.
54. Ostensen M, Brown ND, Chiang PK, et al. Hydroxychloroquine in human breast milk. Eur J Clin Pharmacol 1985;28:357.
55. Akintonwa A, Gbajumo SA, Mabadeje AFB. Placental and mild transfer of chloroquine in humans. Ther Drug Monit 1988;10:147–9.
56. Nation RL, Hackett LP, Dusci LJ, et al. Excretion of hydroxychloroquine in human milk [letter]. Br J Clin Pharmacol 1984;17:368–9.
57. Ette EI, Essien EE, Ogonor JI, et al. Chloroquine in human milk. J Clin Pharmacol 1987;27:499–502.
58. Law I, Ilett KF, Hackett LP, et al. Transfer of chloroquine and desethylchloroquine across the placenta and into milk in Melanesian mothers. Br J Clin Pharmacol 2008;65:674–9.
59. Motta M, Tincani A, Faden D, et al. Follow-up of infants exposed to hydroxychloroquine given to mothers during pregnancy and lactation. J Perinatol 2005;25: 86–9.
60. Esbjorner E, Jarnerot G, Wranne L. Sulphasalazine and sulphpyridine serum levels in children to mothers treated with sulphasalazine during pregnancy and lactation. Acta Paediatr 1987;76:137–42.
61. Jarenerot G, Into-malmberg MB. Sulphasalazine treatemtn durin gbreastfeeding. Scand J Gastroenterol 1979;14:869–71.
62. Berlin CM, Yaffee SJ. Disposition of salicylazosulfapyridine (azulfidine) and metabolites in human breast milk. Dev Pharmacol Ther 1980;1:31–9.
63. Branski D, Kerem E, Gross-Kieselstein E, et al. Bloody diarrhea: a possible complication of sulphasalazine transferred through breast milk. J Pediatr Gastroenterol Nutr 1986;5:316–7.
64. Moretti ME, Verjee Z, Ito S, et al. Breast-feeding during maternal use of azathioprine. Ann Pharmacother 2006;40:2269–72.
65. Sau A, Clarke S, Bass J, et al. Nelson-Piercy. Azathioprine and breastfeeding-is it safe? BJOG 2007;114:498–501.
66. Christensen LA, Dahlerup JF, Nielsen MJ, et al. Azathioprine treatment during lactation. Aliment Pharmacol Ther 2008;28:1209–13.

67. Gardiner SJ, Gearry RB, Roberts RL, et al. Exposure to thiopurine drugs through breast milk is low based on metabolite concentrations in mother-infant pairs. Br J Clin Pharmacol 2006;62:453–6.
68. Nyberg G, Haljamae U, Frisenette-Fich C, et al. Breast-feeding during treatment with cyclosporine. Transplanation 1998;65:253–5.
69. Moretti ME, Sgro M, Johnson DW, et al. Cyclosporine excretion into breast milk. Transplantation 2003;75:2144–6.
70. Jain A, Venkataramanan R, Fung JJ, et al. Pregnancy after liver transplantation under tacrolimus. Transplantation 1997;64:559–65.
71. Gouraud A, Bernard N, Millaret M, et al. Follow-up of tacrolimus breastfed babies. Transplantation 2012;94:e38–40.
72. Johns DG, Rutherford LD, Leighton PC, et al. Secretion of methotrexate into human milk. Am J Obstet Gynecol 1972;112:978–80.
73. Thorne JC, Nadarajah T, Moretti M, et al. Methotrexate use in a breastfeeding patient with rheumatoid arthritis. J Rheumatol 2014;41:2332.
74. Duncan JH, Colvin OM, Fenselau C. Mass spectrometric study of the distribution of cyclophosphamide in humans. Toxicol Appl Pharmacol 1973;24:317–23.
75. Amato D, Niblett JS. Neutropenia from cyclophosphamide in breast milk. Med J Aust 1977;1:383–4.
76. Durodola JI. Administration of cyclophosphamide during late pregnancy and early lactation: a case report. J Natl Med Assoc 1979;71:165–6.
77. Murashima A, Watanabe N, Ozawa N, et al. Etanercept during pregnancy and lactation in a patient with rheumatoid arthritis: drug levels in maternal serum, cord blood, breast milk and the infant's serum. Ann Rheum Dis 2009;68:1793–4.
78. Berthelsen BG, Fjeldsoe-Nielsen H, Nielsen CT, et al. Etanercept concentrations in maternal serum, umbilical cord serum, breast milk and child serum during breastfeeding. Rheumatology 2010;49:2225–7.
79. Keeling S, Wolbink GJ. Measuring multiple etanercept levels in the breast milk of a nursing mother with rheumatoid arthritis. J Rheumatol 2010;37:1551.
80. Ben-Horin S, Yavzori M, Katz L, et al. Adalimumab level in breast milk of a nursing mother. Clin Gastroenterol Hepatol 2010;8:475–6.
81. Fritzsche J, Pilch A, Mury D, et al. Infliximab and adalimumab use during breast-feeding. J Clin Gastroenterol 2012;46:718–9.
82. Julsgaard M, Brown S, Gibson P, et al. Adalimumab levels in an infant. J Crohns Colitis 2013;7:597–8.
83. Vasiliauskas EA, Church JA, Silverman N, et al. Case report: evidence for transplacental transfer of maternally administered infliximab to the newborn. Clin Gastroenterol Hepatol 2006;4:1255–8.
84. Stengel JZ, Arnold HL. Is infliximab safe to use while breastfeeding? World J Gastroenterol 2008;14:3085–7.
85. Kane S, Ford J, Cohen R, et al. Absence of infliximab in infants and breast milk from nursing mothers receiving therapy for Crohn's disease before and after delivery. J Clin Gastroenterol 2009;43:613–6.
86. Forger F, Zbinden A, Villiger PM. Certolizumab treatment during late pregnancy in patients with rheumatic diseases: low drug levels in cord blood but possible risk for maternal infections. A case series of 13 patients. Joint Bone Spine 2016;83:341–3.
87. Martin PL, Oneda S, Treacy G. Effects of an anti-TNFa mooclonal antibody, administered throughout pregnancy and lactation, on the development of the macaque immune system. Am J Reprod Immunol 2007;58:138–49.

88. Nakajima K, Watanabe O, Mochizuki M, et al. Pregnancy outcomes after exposure to tocilizumab: a retrospective analysis of 61 patients in Japan. Mod Rheumatol 2016;26:1–6.
89. Buescher ES, Malinowska I. Soluble receptors and cytokine antagonists in human milk. Pediatr Res 1996;40:839–44.
90. Berger CT, Recher M, Steiner U, et al. A patient's wish: anakinra in pregnancy. Ann Rheum Dis 2009;68:1794–5.
91. Palmeira P, Costa-Carvalho BT, Arslanian C, et al. Transfer of antibodies across the placenta and in breast milk from mothers on intravenous immunoglobulin. Pediatr Allergy Immunol 2009;20:528–35.
92. Achiron A, Kishner I, Dolev M, et al. Effect of intravenous immunoglobulin treatment on pregnancy and postpartum-related relapses in multiple sclerosis. J Neurol 2004;251:1133–7.
93. Huttunen K, Gronhagen-Riska C, Fyhrquist F. Enalapril treatment of a nursing mother with slightly impaired renal function [letter]. Clin Nephrol 1989;31:278.
94. Redman CW, Kelly JG, Cooper WD. The excretion of enalapril and enalaprilat in human breast milk. Eur J Clin Pharmacol 1990;38:99.
95. Devlin RG, Fleiss PM. Captopril in human blood and breast milk. J Clin Pharmacol 1981;21:110–3.
96. Saito I, Takeshita E, Hayashi S, et al. Effect of captopril on plasma prolactin in patients with essential hypertension. Angiology 1990;41(5):377–81.
97. Barrett ME, Heller MM, Stone HF, et al. Raynaud phenomenon of the nipple in breastfeeding mothers: an underdiagnosed cause of nipple pain. JAMA Dermatol 2013;149:300–6.
98. Ehrenkranz RA, Ackerman BA, Hulse JD. Nifedipine transfer into human milk. J Pediatr 1989;114:478–80.
99. Orme ML, Lewis PJ, De Swiet M, et al. May mothers given warfarin breast-feed their infants? Br Med J 1977;1:1564–5.
100. Schindler D, Graham TP. Warfarin overdose in a breast-feeding woman. West J Emerg Med 2011;12:216–7.
101. Guillonneau M, de Crepy A, Aufrant C, et al. Breast-feeding is possible in case of maternal treatment with enoxaparin. Arch Pediatr (Paris) 1996;3:513–4 [in French].
102. Ben-Chetrit E, Scherrmann JM, Levy M. Colchicine in breast milk of patients with familial Mediterranean fever. Arthritis Rheum 1996;39:1213–7.
103. Guillonneau M, Aigrain EJ, Galliot M, et al. Colchicine is excreted at high concentrations in human breast milk [letter]. Eur J Obstet Gynecol Reprod Biol 1995;61:177–8.

Outcomes in Children Born to Women with Rheumatic Diseases

Évelyne Vinet, MD, PhD[a,b,*], Sasha Bernatsky, MD, PhD[a,b]

KEYWORDS

- Systemic lupus erythematosus • Rheumatoid arthritis • Pregnancy • Children
- Long-term outcomes

KEY POINTS

- Genetic factors and in utero exposure to maternal autoantibodies, cytokines, and medications, as well as obstetric complications, might predispose SLE and RA offspring to adverse health outcomes.
- Children born to women with SLE and RA are potentially at increased risk of neurodevelopmental disorders, congenital heart defects, and autoimmune diseases, compared with children from the general population.
- Although clinicians should probably be aware of this increased relative risk of adverse health outcomes, the absolute risk is small and women with SLE and RA should not be discouraged from having children.

INTRODUCTION

Systemic lupus erythematosus (SLE) and rheumatoid arthritis (RA) are the most prevalent autoimmune rheumatic diseases, and predominantly occur in women during childbearing years. To date, research has mainly focused on assessing the risk of immediate complications during SLE and RA pregnancies, with studies documenting a higher risk of adverse obstetric outcomes, such as preterm births and infants small for gestational age (SGA). However, until recently, little was known regarding the long-term health of children born to affected women. SLE and RA offspring are potentially exposed in utero to maternal autoantibodies, cytokines, and drugs, as well as

Disclosures: Fonds de Recherche en Santé du Québec (FRQS) Junior 1 Salary Award (E. Vinet); FRQS Career Award (S. Bernatsky).
[a] Division of Clinical Epidemiology, McGill University Health Centre, Pine Avenue, Montreal, Québec H3A 1A1, Canada; [b] Division of Rheumatology, McGill University Health Centre, Cedar Avenue, Montreal, Québec H3G 1A4, Canada
* Corresponding author. Montreal General Hospital, McGill University Health Center, 1650 Cedar Avenue, Room A6 162.2, Montreal, Québec H3G 1A4, Canada.
E-mail address: evelyne.vinet@mcgill.ca

obstetric complications. This might result in developmental anomalies, congenital defects, and/or disease susceptibility. In the past few years, observational studies have suggested an increased risk of adverse health outcomes, including neurodevelopmental disorders, congenital heart defects (CHDs), hematological malignancies, and autoimmune diseases, in offspring born to mothers with SLE and RA. We present a review of the current evidence regarding the risk of adverse health outcomes in SLE and RA offspring, as well as potential mechanisms involved in their pathogenesis.

Neurodevelopmental Disorders

Epidemiologic data suggest that children born to women with SLE may have an increased risk of neurodevelopmental disorders compared with children born to healthy women. Several retrospective studies suggest that children, particularly sons, of mothers with SLE are at increased risk (up to 25%–45%) for learning disabilities.[1–3] In a small retrospective study using parental report, the prevalence of learning problems in offspring of mothers with SLE was more than twice that reported for controls.[2] A prospective study assessed the neurodevelopment of 57 children born to mothers with SLE and 49 controls using standardized tests.[4] Offspring of mothers with SLE had more than a threefold increase in anomalies related to learning and memory, as well as behavior. In a retrospective cohort study of 60 SLE offspring, in utero exposure to azathioprine conferred more than a sixfold increased risk of having special educational needs (used as a proxy for developmental delays), when adjusting for disease severity and obstetric complications.[5]

Although these previous studies support the hypothesis of an increased risk of neurodevelopmental disorders in offspring of mothers with SLE, the studies were marked by important methodological limitations: all had limited sample size; only one controlled for obstetric complications and medication exposures; and most used parental report, did not include a control group, and/or were retrospective in nature.

In 2015, investigators reported data from the Offspring of SLE Mothers Registry (OSLER), a large population-based cohort using Quebec's health care databases and including 719 children born to mothers with SLE, and a matched control group of 8493 children born to unaffected mothers.[6] SLE offspring were more frequently found to have a diagnosis of autism spectrum disorders (ASD) compared with unexposed children (frequency of recorded ASDs 1.4% [95% confidence interval (95% CI) 0.8–2.5] vs 0.6% [95% CI 0.5–0.8]), a difference of 0.8% (95% CI 0.1–1.9). The mean age at ASD diagnosis was younger in offspring of mothers with SLE (mean 3.8 years, 95% CI 1.8–5.8) compared with offspring of controls (mean 5.7 years, 95% CI 4.9–6.5). In multivariate analysis accounting for maternal characteristics and obstetric complications, SLE offspring had a substantially increased risk of ASD compared with controls (odds ratio [OR] 2.19, 95% CI 1.09–4.39). The younger age at ASD diagnosis could suggest either more severe cases or increased surveillance within the SLE population.

In addition to cohort evidence of an increased risk of neurodevelopmental disorders in offspring of mothers with SLE, numerous case-control studies have suggested an increased prevalence of SLE and other autoimmune diseases in mothers of children affected with neurodevelopmental disorders.[7–9] In a case-control study of 61 children with ASD and 46 healthy controls, affected children had more than an eightfold increase in the odds of having a mother with an autoimmune disorder (by self-report) than unaffected children.[9] SLE was observed in 13% of children with ASD, versus 4% of healthy controls. Another large population-based study showed similar results.[7] In this study, children with ASD were more likely than unaffected children to have a mother diagnosed with an autoimmune rheumatic disease (relative risk 1.56, 95% CI 1.08, 2.17), whereas the likelihood of having a father with these diseases did not differ. This suggests that the association between SLE and neurodevelopmental disorders might be influenced by prenatal exposure to maternal antibodies and/or fetal environment during gestation.

Limited evidence suggests a potentially increased risk of neurodevelopmental disorders in RA offspring, as shown by a recent systematic literature review[10] that identified only 2 observational studies assessing this issue.[7,9] In one study,[7] 46% of ASD offspring had a first-degree relative with RA compared with 26% of controls ($P = .04$). Moreover, in a population-based study including 3325 children with ASD and more than 650,000 controls, investigators observed an increased risk of ASD in children with a maternal RA compared with children born to unaffected mothers (OR 1.70, 95% CI 1.07–2.54).[9] These observational studies are marked by important methodological limitations; study effect estimates were relatively imprecise, it is unclear to what extent the subjects represented the population base, neither controlled for medication exposures, and only one accounted for obstetric complications and considered the timing of RA diagnosis in relation to the pregnancy.

In utero exposure to maternal immunoglobulin G (IgG) antibodies is increasingly recognized as an important environmental risk factor for neurodevelopmental disorders. Maternal IgG antibodies begin to cross the placenta during the second trimester of pregnancy, reaching circulating levels in the newborn that exceed maternal levels due to active transport across the placenta.[11] In the presence of maternal autoimmunity, autoantibodies also cross the placenta and can interfere with fetal development. Although offending maternal autoantibodies are cleared from the child's circulation within the first 6 months of life, autoantibody-mediated injury in utero can result in long-term damage to organs (eg, congenital heart block in neonatal lupus).[12]

The blood-brain barrier blocks IgG entry into the adult central nervous system (CNS), but in the fetus, the immature blood-brain barrier allows IgG access to the developing brain.[11] Genetic predisposition may increase susceptibility to neurodevelopmental disorders in children exposed in utero to offending maternal IgG.[13] Antibodies directed against fetal brain proteins (yet to be identified) have been observed in 10% to 12% of mothers of children with ASD.[11] This antibody reactivity has been shown to be absent in mothers of normally developing children. When human maternal fetal brain-reactive antibodies from mothers of children with ASD were administered to pregnant mice, behavioral alterations in the offspring were noted.[14] In this mouse model, an increased number of microglial cells were observed in the brain of exposed offspring, suggesting that these brain-reactive antibodies may mediate their effects through inflammatory changes.[14]

Diamond and colleagues[15] recently showed that 53% of mothers of a child with ASD with fetal brain-reactive antibodies also exhibited anti-nuclear autoantibodies compared with 13% of mothers with ASD without fetal brain-reactive antibodies and 15% of control women. They also observed an increased prevalence of autoimmune diseases in mothers with ASD with fetal brain-reactive antibodies. Mothers with ASD with fetal brain-reactive antibodies were 3 times more likely to have SLE and RA compared with mothers of a child with ASD without these antibodies and control women of childbearing age, suggesting that a subset of ASD may be related to in utero maternal antibody exposure.

New experimental data further support a potential link between in utero exposure to SLE and neurodevelopmental disorders. A subset of anti-double-stranded DNA antibodies, anti–N-methyl-D-aspartate receptor (NMDAR) antibodies, are present in up to 60% of women with SLE. In a murine model, these antibodies have been shown to cross the placenta, induce fetal brain neuronal apoptosis, and cause cognitive impairments in offspring, preferentially in male individuals.[16,17] Affected offspring displayed smaller-sized neocortical neurons and neuronal migration defects, findings observed in histologic studies of humans affected with learning disabilities.[18]

It is noteworthy that pregnant mice exposed to anti-NMDAR antibodies had a marked preferential loss of female fetuses, resulting in an increased male-to-female ratio in their offspring.[16] Interestingly, investigators have recently demonstrated that mothers with SLE had substantially increased odds of having male offspring compared with mothers without SLE (OR 1.18, 95% CI 1.01–1.38).[19] This finding mirrors experimental data and parallels the male predominance seen in neurodevelopmental disorders.

Other autoantibodies found in SLE may also potentially alter fetal brain development. Antiphospholipid antibodies (aPL), present in 30% of women with SLE (and 15% of subjects with RA), have been found at high levels in the serum of exposed neonates.[20] These antibodies can bind CNS cells and, in murine models, prolonged exposure to aPL induces hyperactive behavior and neurologic dysfunction.[21,22] In theory, aPL might be implicated in inducing neurodevelopmental disorders in children born to women with SLE.

Maternal cytokines may reach the fetal circulation,[23] and the maternal cytokine milieu might constitute an another important environmental risk factor. Interleukin-6 (IL-6) is known for its primordial role in brain development[24]: administration in pregnant mice caused substantial behavioral and social deficits in the offspring, whereas coadministration with an anti–IL-6 antibody prevented these deficits.[24] IL-6 is involved in autoantibody production in RA and SLE, and affected patients have markedly elevated IL-6 blood levels.[25] IL-6 could have a direct effect on the fetal brain or enhance the production of maternal fetal brain-reactive antibodies, which could cross-react with the fetal brain, leading to neurodevelopmental disorders.

Recently, maternal IL-17a has been identified as a potentially critical cytokine in the development of ASD in offspring. Rodents subjected to maternal immune activation (MIA) develop ASD phenotypes. In a mouse model, Choi and colleagues[26] showed that T-helper 17 (TH17) cells and the effector cytokine IL-17a are required in mothers for MIA-induced behavioral abnormalities in offspring. MIA induced abnormal cortical development in the fetal brain, which was dependent on maternal IL-17a; treatment with anti–IL-17a antibodies in the pregnant mothers improved both behavioral abnormalities and abnormal cortical development in offspring.

Genes implicated in autoimmune disorders, including SLE and RA are significantly more prevalent in subjects with ASD.[23] One such gene is the C4B null allele, strongly associated with SLE.[27] Of particular interest, the C4B null allele is 4 times more common in individuals with ASD compared with controls.[28] As presence of the C4B null allele leads to partial C4B deficiency, and because the complement system is involved in brain tissue remodeling and repair, alterations in C4B levels might alter the fetal immune response to in utero immunologic insults, resulting in pathologic changes.[29]

Subjects with both RA and ASD share a common genetic predisposition to HLA-DRB1*04 alleles.[30–32] The association with the HLA-DRB1*04 alleles represents the firmest link between a genetic susceptibility factor and RA, conferring up to an 11-fold increase in RA risk.[30,31] Previous case-control studies have consistently shown increased frequency of HLA-DRB1*04 in ASD offspring and their mothers, but not their fathers.[32] In a recent study assessing transmission disequilibrium of the HLA-DRB1*04 alleles in 31 families of ASD offspring, investigators observed significant transmission disequilibrium for HLADRB1*04 (OR 4.67, 95% CI 1.34–16.24) from maternal grandparents to mothers of ASD cases, whereas they did not observe HLA-DRB1*04 transmission from mothers or fathers to offspring with ASD.[32] These findings support a role for HLA-DRB1*04 as an ASD risk factor acting in mothers during pregnancy (ie, not due to genetic transmission from parents, but potentially through maternal action in utero), raising the possibility of a maternal immune component to ASD pathogenesis.

Finally, SLE and RA pregnancies are at increased risk of adverse obstetric outcomes, such as prematurity and SGA, which are potential risk factors for neurodevelopmental disorders.[33–35] Observational studies report a 1.5 to 3.0-fold increase in neurodevelopmental disorders in children born preterm or SGA versus controls.[36,37] Thus, obstetric complications in women with SLE and RA may also increase neurodevelopmental disorders in offspring.

Congenital Heart Defects

CHDs are the most frequent type of birth defects, accounting for approximately a third of all congenital anomalies[38]; they are associated with substantial childhood morbidity.[39] In utero exposures, such as maternal illness and medications, are thought to play an important role in the yet to be fully elucidated etiology of CHD.[40] In particular, a recent study suggests a threefold increased risk of CHD in children born to mothers with various systemic autoimmune rheumatic diseases[41]; however, the investigators did not specifically assess the SLE and RA effect estimates for risk and did not control for medication exposures.

Until recently, very few uncontrolled observational studies had assessed CHD in offspring of mothers with SLE. Notably, in a study of fetal echocardiography in a small number of SLE pregnancies,[42] 7.5% of fetuses had a CHD, which is more than fivefold greater than that observed among live births from the general population (0.6%–1.3%).[43] After excluding cases with CHD that could have caused congenital heart block, investigators observed CHD in 16% to 42% of children with congenital heart block born to mothers with anti-Ro/SSA antibodies.[44–48] The most frequently observed CHDs were atrial septal defects, ventricular septal defects (VSD), and valve anomalies.[44–48]

In 2015, Vinet and colleagues[6] assessed the risk of CHD in SLE offspring within the large population-based OSLER cohort. In comparison with unexposed children, SLE offspring experienced more CHD (5.2% [95% CI 3.7–7.1] vs 1.9% [95% CI 1.6–2.2], difference 3.3% [95% CI 1.9–5.2]). In multivariable analyses, children born to women with SLE had a substantially increased risk of CHD (OR 2.62, 95% CI 1.77–3.88) compared with unexposed children. Subgroup analyses accounting for medication exposures were similar. In addition, offspring of mothers with SLE had a substantially increased risk of having a CHD repair procedure (OR 5.82, 95% CI 1.77–19.09). These data suggest that SLE offspring are at increased risk of CHD, and at least part of this risk might be independent of in utero medication exposures.

Data are more limited regarding the risk of CHD in RA offspring. In a large cohort study using Quebec's administrative data (n = 8810), investigators observed a substantially increased risk of CHD in children born to women diagnosed with RA during childhood compared with children from the general population (OR 2.09, 95% CI 1.23–3.55).[49] A CHD diagnosis was documented in 1.2% of RA offspring (95% CI 0.69–1.71) as opposed to 0.6% of control children (95% CI 0.42–0.78). Although analyses were limited by the lack of drug information, these findings suggest that RA offspring might also be at increased risk of CHD.

Maternal SLE/RA-related mechanisms that could be implicated in the physiopathology of CHD in offspring include autoantibody-mediated damage and cytokine imbalance. Anti-Ro/SSA and anti-La/SSB antibodies, found in, respectively, 40% and 20% of women with SLE and RA, cross the placenta and are associated with development of neonatal lupus, with congenital heart block being the most characteristic cardiac manifestation. Investigators have demonstrated that maternal anti-Ro/SSA and anti-La/SSB antibodies bind apoptotic fetal cardiocytes, resulting in the release of proinflammatory and profibrosing cytokines, and, ultimately, scarring.[50]

This process likely extends beyond the conduction tissue, involving the myocardium, endocardium, and valves. In a recent retrospective analysis of autopsies from 18 cardiac neonatal lupus cases, cardiac histologic damage outside of the conduction system was frequently observed.[47] Six (40%) of 15 of deaths due to congenital heart block had pathology findings, such as fibrosis and calcification of the valves and/or valve apparatus.[47]

Cardiac septation occurs early in embryogenesis and is complete by 6 weeks' gestation.[51] Because transplacental passage of maternal autoantibodies occurs later (beginning at approximately 16 weeks), it is unlikely that maternal autoantibodies directly interfere. However, muscular VSDs, which account for 75% of all VSDs, are thought to arise from foci of cellular death during active cardiac remodeling within an already formed ventricular septum.[52] In addition, maternal autoantibodies might prevent closure of cardiac septal defects that might have closed naturally, possibly explaining the excess risk of cardiac septal defects in offspring of mothers with SLE.

aPL antibodies also cross the placenta: in one recent study, 40% of neonates born to women with antiphospholipid syndrome had positive aPL in cord blood.[20] In aPL-positive adult patients with and without SLE, aPLs are strongly associated with valvular disease,[53] and valvular deposits of aPL are thought to play an important pathogenic role.[53] Although prior studies have reported perinatal thrombotic events occurring in children born to aPL-positive mothers, there are no data on the prevalence of congenital valve anomalies or other types of CHD in these children[54]; in theory, however, transplacental aPL could play a role in valve anomalies in exposed fetuses.

Cytokines, such as transforming growth factor beta (TGF-beta), play an important role in cardiac embryogenesis. In particular, adequate endocardial cushion formation, which is a critical step in cardiac septation, requires appropriate expression of TGF-beta.[55] Defective levels of TGF-beta have been associated with CHD in animal models, whereas high levels have been linked to CHD in human studies.[55–57] Serum levels of TGF-beta-1 are substantially lower in subjects with SLE (inversely correlating with disease activity), whereas they are higher in subjects with RA (correlating with disease activity).[54,58,59] Because transplacental transfer of circulating TGF-beta can occur from mother to fetus, abnormal levels of maternal TGF-beta might alter normal fetal heart development, potentially leading to an increased risk of CHD.

Hematological Malignancies

Hematologic malignancies, such as leukemia and lymphoma, account for approximately 40% of new cancer diagnoses in children, with an incidence of up to 12 cases per 100,000 annually.[60] Diffuse large B-cell lymphoma (DLBCL), a non-Hodgkin lymphoma, is one of the most common lymphomas among children and adolescents, representing 20% and 40% of new lymphoma cases in children and adolescents, respectively.[60]

Patients with SLE and RA have an increased risk of hematological malignancies, particularly non-Hodgkin lymphoma, compared with the general population.[58] Large population-based studies have consistently shown more than a twofold increase in the risk of leukemia and lymphoma in SLE and RA, thought to be due to chronic immune stimulation.[58] The most common type of hematological malignancy in SLE and RA is DLBCL.

Data on hematological malignancies in RA offspring are very limited, and such data are nonexistent in SLE. In one cohort study, mothers with RA had an increased risk of having a child with lymphoma or leukemia compared with general population rates (relative risk 1.7, 95% CI 0.9–2.8).[61] In another cohort study of offspring born to RA parents, there was a substantially increased risk of Hodgkin's lymphoma (standardized incidence ratio 3.2, 95% CI 1.0–7.4)[62]; however, the investigators did not provide a specific estimate for offspring born to mothers with RA, as opposed to fathers with RA. In addition, in both studies, no attention was paid to the timing of RA diagnosis in relation to the pregnancy.

As childhood hematological cancers are thought to arise from an aberrant immune response, genetic studies have investigated the potential role of genes involved in the immune system. Notably, several investigators have reported an association between HLA-DRB1*04 alleles and a twofold increase in the risk of acute lymphoblastic leukemia in children.[63] Thus, offspring of subjects with RA might be at increased risk of hematological malignancies through inheritance of risk alleles.

Rheumatic and Nonrheumatic Autoimmune Diseases

Several studies have suggested a familial aggregation of SLE and RA, as well as several autoimmune diseases, such as type 1 diabetes. However, only 2 studies have specifically assessed the risk of autoimmune diseases in offspring born to mothers with SLE or RA. Preliminary findings from the OSLER cohort showed a potentially twofold increase in the risk of nonrheumatic autoimmune diseases (including type 1 diabetes and inflammatory bowel diseases) in children born to women with SLE compared with children from the general population.[64] However, the effect estimate for the risk of rheumatic autoimmune diseases was inconclusive.

In a large Danish population-based study of 13,566 RA offspring, Rom and colleagues[65] studied children whose mothers had RA and compared them with children whose mothers did not have RA. In RA offspring, there was higher morbidity for 8/11 International Classification of Diseases groups. Similar results were observed in 6330 children whose fathers had RA. The investigators reported a substantial increase in the risk of specific rheumatic and nonrheumatic autoimmune diseases with up to a threefold increase in the risk of juvenile idiopathic arthritis (hazard ratio [HR] for maternal RA 3.30 [95% CI 2.71–4.03] and for paternal RA 2.97 [95% CI 2.20–4.01]), an increased risk of up to 40% of type 1 diabetes (HR for maternal RA 1.37 [95% CI 1.12–1.66] and for paternal RA 1.44 [95% CI 1.09–1.90]), and up to a 30% increased risk of asthma (HR for maternal RA 1.28 [95% CI 1.20–1.36] and for paternal RA 1.15 [95% CI 1.04–1.26]). As an increased risk of autoimmune diseases was found both in children exposed to maternal RA and children exposed to paternal RA, genetic factors are likely to play an important role, although this was not specifically studied by the investigators.

Interestingly, in the previously described study, increased risk of infectious diseases as well as mental and behavioral disorders were seen only in offspring exposed to maternal RA (the investigators did not provide a specific risk estimate for neurodevelopmental disorders). In addition, stronger associations were observed in children born to mothers with RA compared with children born to fathers with RA. Thus, fetal programming, through in utero exposures to maternal autoantibodies, cytokines, drugs, and obstetric complications, might all have an etiologic role in certain adverse health outcomes in offspring.

SUMMARY

Children born to women with SLE and RA are potentially at increased risk of adverse health outcomes, including neurodevelopmental disorders, CHDs, hematological malignancies, and autoimmune diseases. It is important to stress that the absolute risk of these adverse health outcomes is quite small, occurring in only a very limited numbers of offspring. Clearly most offspring born to mothers with RA or SLE will not be affected. Thus, although clinicians may use data from published studies when counseling women with RA or SLE who are concerned about these risks, most women with

SLE or RA (barring specific medical complications) should not be discouraged from planning a pregnancy. Absolute risks may be more relevant than relative risks when counseling prospective parents.

Further research is needed to fully elucidate the potential disease-related factors that might lead to the increased risk of adverse health outcomes in offspring, as well as to guide the optimal monitoring of SLE and RA offspring. This will allow more personalized counseling for women with SLE or RA contemplating pregnancy, and may even guide eventual trials of interventions for subgroups of women at greatest risk.

REFERENCES

1. Lahita RG. Systemic lupus erythematosus: learning disability in the male offspring of female patients and relationship to laterality. Psychoneuroendocrinology 1988; 13(5):385–96.
2. McAllister DL, Kaplan BJ, Edworthy SM, et al. The influence of systemic lupus erythematosus on fetal development: cognitive, behavioral, and health trends. J Int Neuropsychol Soc 1997;3(4):370–6.
3. Ross G, Sammaritano L, Nass R, et al. Effects of mothers' autoimmune disease during pregnancy on learning disabilities and hand preference in their children. Arch Pediatr Adolesc Med 2003;157(4):397–402.
4. Urowitz MB, Gladman DD, MacKinnon A, et al. Neurocognitive abnormalities in offspring of mothers with systemic lupus erythematosus. Lupus 2008;17(6): 555–60.
5. Marder W, Ganser MA, Romero V, et al. In utero azathioprine exposure and increased utilization of special educational services in children born to mothers with systemic lupus erythematosus. Arthritis Care Res (Hoboken) 2013;65(5): 759–66.
6. Vinet É, Pineau CA, Clarke AE, et al. Increased risk of congenital heart defects in children born to women with systemic lupus erythematosus: results from the OSLER study. Circulation 2015;131(2):149–56.
7. Comi AM, Zimmerman AW, Frye VH, et al. Familial clustering of autoimmune disorders and evaluation of medical risk factors in autism. J Child Neurol 1999;14: 388–94.
8. Sweeten TL, Bowyer SL, Posey DJ, et al. Increased prevalence of familial autoimmunity in probands with pervasive developmental disorders. Pediatrics 2003; 112(5):e420.
9. Atladóttir HO, Pedersen MG, Thorsen P, et al. Association of family history of autoimmune diseases and autism spectrum disorders. Pediatr 2009;124:687–94.
10. Wojcik S, Bernatsky S, Platt R, et al. Risk of autism spectrum disorders in children born to mothers with rheumatoid arthritis: a systematic literature review. J Rheumatol 2015;42(Suppl 7):1263–351 [abstract: 72].
11. Braunschweig D, Van de Water J. Maternal autoantibodies in autism. Arch Neurol 2012;69(6):693–9.
12. Brucato A, Frassi M, Franceschini F, et al. Risk of complete congenital heart block in newborns of mothers with anti-Ro/SSA antibodies detected by counterimmunoelectrophoresis. Arthritis Rheum 2001;44:1832–5.
13. Benayed R, Gharani N, Rossman I, et al. Support for the homeobox transcription factor gene ENGRAILED 2 as an autism spectrum disorder susceptibility locus. Am J Hum Genet 2005;77(5):851–68.

14. Singer HS, Morris C, Gause C, et al. Prenatal exposure to antibodies from mothers of children with autism produces neurobehavioral alterations: a pregnant dam mouse model. J Neuroimmunol 2009;211(1–2):39–48.

15. Brimberg L, Sadiq A, Gregersen PK, et al. Brain-reactive IgG correlates with autoimmunity in mothers of a child with an autism spectrum disorder. Mol Psychiatry 2013;18(11):1171–7.

16. Wang L, Zhou D, Lee J, et al. Female mouse fetal loss mediated by maternal autoantibody. J Exp Med 2012;209(6):1083–9.

17. Lee JY, Huerta PT, Zhang J, et al. Neurotoxic autoantibodies mediate congenital cortical impairment of offspring in maternal lupus. Nat Med 2009;15(1):91–6.

18. Nopoulos P, Berg S, Castellenos FX, et al. Developmental brain anomalies in children with attention-deficit hyperactivity disorder. J Child Neurol 2000;15(2):102–8.

19. Vinet E, Bernatsky S, Pineau CA, et al. Increased male-to-female ratio in children born to women with systemic lupus erythematosus. Arthritis Rheum 2013;65(4):1129.

20. Mekinian A, Lachassinne E, Nicaise-Roland P, et al. European registry of babies born to mothers with antiphospholipid syndrome. Ann Rheum Dis 2013;72(2):217–22.

21. Caronti B, Calderaro C, Alessandri C, et al. Serum anti-beta2-glycoprotein I antibodies from patients with antiphospholipid antibody syndrome bind central nervous system cells. J Autoimmun 1998;11:425–9.

22. Shrot S, Katzav A, Korczyn AD, et al. Behavioral and cognitive deficits occur only after prolonged exposure of mice to antiphospholipid antibodies. Lupus 2002;11:736–43.

23. Sperner-Unterweger B. Immunological aetiology of major psychiatric disorders: evidence and therapeutic implications. Drugs 2005;65(11):1493–520.

24. Smith SE, Li J, Garbett K, et al. Maternal immune activation alters fetal brain development through interleukin-6. J Neurosci 2007;27(40):10695–702.

25. Tsokos GC. Systemic lupus erythematosus. N Engl J Med 2011;365(22):2110–21.

26. Choi GB, Yim YS, Wong H, et al. The maternal interleukin-17a pathway in mice promotes autism-like phenotypes in offspring. Science 2016;351(6276):933–9.

27. Naves M, Hajeer AH, Teh LS, et al. Complement C4B null allele status confers risk for systemic lupus erythematosus in a Spanish population. Eur J Immunogenet 1998;25(4):317–20.

28. Warren RP, Singh VK, Averett RE, et al. Immunogenetic studies in autism and related disorders. Mol Chem Neuropathol 1996;28(1–3):77–81.

29. Odell D, Maciulis A, Cutler A, et al. Confirmation of the association of the C4B null allelle in autism. Hum Immunol 2005;66(2):140–5.

30. Fries JF, Wolfe F, Apple R, et al. HLA-DRB1 genotype associations in 793 white patients from a rheumatoid arthritis inception cohort: frequency, severity, and treatment bias. Arthritis Rheum 2002;46(9):2320–9.

31. de Vries RR, Huizinga TW, Toes RE. Redefining the HLA and RA association: to be or not to be anti-CCP positive. J Autoimmun 2005;25(Suppl):21–5.

32. Johnson WG, Buyske S, Mars AE, et al. HLA-DR4 as a risk allele for autism acting in mothers of probands possibly during pregnancy. Arch Pediatr Adolesc Med 2009;163(6):542–6.

33. Cortes-Hernandes J, Ordi-Ros J, Paredes F, et al. Clinical predictors of fetal and maternal outcome in systemic lupus erythematosus: a prospective study of 103 pregnancies. Rheumatology 2002;41:643–50.

34. Petri M, Allbriton J. Fetal outcome of lupus pregnancy: a retrospective case-control study of the Hopkins lupus cohort. J Rheumatol 1993;20:650–6.

35. Molad Y, Borkowski T, Monselise A, et al. Maternal and fetal outcome of lupus pregnancy: a prospective study of 29 pregnancies. Lupus 2005;14:145–51.

36. Thapar A, Cooper M, Jefferies R, et al. What causes attention deficit hyperactivity disorder? Arch Dis Child 2012;97(3):260–5.

37. Lampi KM, Lehtonen L, Tran PL, et al. Risk of autism spectrum disorders in low birth weight and small for gestational age infants. J Pediatr 2012;161(5):830–6.

38. Canfield MA, Honein MA, Yuskiv N, et al. National estimates and race/ethnic-specific variation of selected birth defects in the United States, 1999-2001. Birth Defects Res A Clin Mol Teratol 2006;76(11):747–56.

39. Talner CN. Report of the New England Regional Infant Cardiac Program, by Donald C. Fyler, MD, Pediatrics, 1980;65(suppl):375–461. Pediatrics 1998;102(1 Pt 2): 258–9.

40. Williams LJ, Correa A, Rasmussen S. Maternal lifestyle factors and risk for ventricular septal defects. Birth Defects Res A Clin Mol Teratol 2004;70:59–64.

41. Liu S, Joseph KS, Lisonkova S, et al, Canadian Perinatal Surveillance System (Public Health Agency of Canada). Association between maternal chronic conditions and congenital heart defects: a population-based cohort study. Circulation 2013;128(6):583–9.

42. Krishnan AN, Sable CA, Donofrio MT. Spectrum of fetal echocardiographic findings in fetuses of women with clinical or serologic evidence of systemic lupus erythematosus. J Matern Fetal Neonatal Med 2008;21(11):776–82.

43. Hoffman JI, Kaplan S. The incidence of congenital heart disease. J Am Coll Cardiol 2002;39:1890–900.

44. Costedoat-Chalumeau N, Amoura Z, Villain E, et al. Anti-SSA/Ro antibodies and the heart: more than complete congenital heart block? A review of electrocardiographic and myocardial abnormalities and of treatment options. Arthritis Res Ther 2005;7(2):69–73.

45. Costedoat-Chalumeau N, Amoura Z, Lupoglazoff JM, et al. Outcome of pregnancies in patients with anti-SSA/Ro antibodies: a study of 165 pregnancies, with special focus on electrocardiographic variations in the children and comparison with a control group. Arthritis Rheum 2004;50(10):3187–94.

46. Buyon JP, Hiebert R, Copel J, et al. Autoimmune-associated congenital heart block: demographics, mortality, morbidity and recurrence rates obtained from a national neonatal lupus registry. J Am Coll Cardiol 1998;31(7):1658–66.

47. Llanos C, Friedman DM, Saxena A, et al. Anatomical and pathological findings in hearts from fetuses and infants with cardiac manifestations of neonatal lupus. Rheumatology (Oxford) 2012;51(6):1086–92.

48. Davey DL, Bratton SL, Bradley DJ, et al. Relation of maternal anti-Ro/La antibodies to aortic dilation in patients with congenital complete heart block. Am J Cardiol 2011;108(4):561–4.

49. Ehrmann Feldman D, Vinet E, Bernatsky S, et al. Birth outcomes in women with a history of juvenile idiopathic arthritis. J Rheumatol 2016;43(4):804–9.

50. Izmirly PM, Buyon JP, Saxena A. Neonatal lupus: advances in understanding pathogenesis and identifying treatments of cardiac disease. Curr Opin Rheumatol 2012;24(5):466–72.

51. Van Praagh R. Section II - Developmental anatomy, Chapter 2 – embryology. In: Keane JF, Lock JE, Fyler DC, editors. Nadas' pediatric cardiology. 2nd edition. Philadelphia: Saunders (Elsevier); 2006. p. 13–25.

52. Clark EB. Growth, morphogenesis, and function: the dynamics of cardiovascular development. In: Moller JM, Neal WA, editors. Fetal, neonatal, and infant heart disease. 1st edition. New York: Appleton-Century-Crofts; 1989. p. 1–22.
53. Zuily S, Huttin O, Mohamed S, et al. Valvular heart disease in antiphospholipid syndrome. Curr Rheumatol Rep 2013;15(4):320.
54. Boffa MC, Lachassinne E. Infant perinatal thrombosis and antiphospholipid antibodies: a review. Lupus 2007;16:634–41.
55. Arthur HM, Bamforth SD. TGFβ signaling and congenital heart disease: insights from mouse studies. Birth Defects Res A Clin Mol Teratol 2011;91(6):423–34.
56. Wheeler JB, Ikonomidis JS, Jones JA. Connective tissue disorders and cardiovascular complications: the indomitable role of transforming growth factor-beta signaling. Adv Exp Med Biol 2014;802:107–27.
57. Su DL, Lu ZM, Shen MN, et al. Roles of pro- and anti-inflammatory cytokines in the pathogenesis of SLE. J Biomed Biotechnol 2012;2012:347141.
58. Kaiser R. Incidence of lymphoma in patients with rheumatoid arthritis: a systematic review of the literature. Clin Lymphoma Myeloma 2008;8(2):87–93.
59. Baecklund E, Iliadou A, Askling J, et al. Association of chronic inflammation, not its treatment, with increased lymphoma risk in rheumatoid arthritis. Arthritis Rheum 2006;54(3):692–701.
60. Cotterill SJ, Parker L, Malcolm AJ, et al. Incidence and survival for cancer in children and young adults in the North of England, 1968–1995: a report from the Northern Region Young Persons' malignant disease registry. Br J Cancer 2000; 83(3):397–403.
61. Mellemkjær L, Alexander F, Olsen JH. Cancer among children of parents with autoimmune diseases. Br J Cancer 2000;82(7):1353–7.
62. Ekström K, Hjalgrim H, Brandt L, et al. Risk of malignant lymphomas in patients with rheumatoid arthritis and in their first-degree relatives. Arthritis Rheum 2003;48(4):963–70.
63. Urayama KY, Thompson PD, Taylor M, et al. Genetic variation in the extended major histocompatibility complex and susceptibility to childhood acute lymphoblastic leukemia: a review of the evidence. Front Oncol 2013;12(3):345–9.
64. Couture J, Bernatsky S, Scott S, et al. Rheumatic and non-rheumatic autoimmune diseases in SLE offspring. Arthritis Rheum 2015;67(Suppl 10) [abstract: 2125].
65. Rom AL, Wu CS, Olsen J, et al. Parental rheumatoid arthritis and long-term child morbidity: a nationwide cohort study. Ann Rheum Dis 2016;75(10):1831–7.

Infertility – Prevention and Management

Emily C. Somers, PhD, ScM[a,b,c], Wendy Marder, MD, MS[a,b,*]

KEYWORDS

- Infertility • Systemic autoimmune diseases • Fertility preservation

KEY POINTS

- Women with autoimmune diseases have elevated risk for primary ovarian insufficiency, likely resulting from the underlying inflammatory state, alterations of the hypothalamic-pituitary-gonadal (HPG) axis, and medication exposures.
- Increasingly, more options are available for ovarian preservation alongside gonadotoxic treatment regimens, including strategies for minimizing cumulative exposure of alkylating agents, such as cyclophosphamide (CYC), and the use of adjunctive gonadotropin-releasing hormone analog (GnRH-a) therapy.
- Given that early adulthood and mid-adulthood are periods of increasing risk for development of many autoimmune diseases, particular emphasis on reproductive and family planning issues in this population is of upmost importance.

INTRODUCTION

For women with rheumatic autoimmune diseases, including systemic lupus erythematosus (SLE), rheumatoid arthritis, and ankylosing spondylitis, the risk of subfertility and infertility is higher than in the general population. Given that early adulthood and mid-adulthood are periods of increasing risk for development of many autoimmune diseases,[1,2] particular emphasis on reproductive and family planning issues is of upmost importance. For instance, lupus has often been referred to as a disease of women in their childbearing years; the authors have shown that incidence of SLE among black women peaks during ages 25 to 29 years (**Fig. 1**).[3]

Disclosure Statement: The authors have nothing to disclose.
[a] Division of Rheumatology, Department of Internal Medicine, University of Michigan, North Campus Research Complex, B014 G236, 2800 Plymouth Road, SPC 2800, Ann Arbor, MI 48109-2800, USA; [b] Department of Obstetrics and Gynecology, University of Michigan, North Campus Research Complex, B014 G236, 2800 Plymouth Road, SPC 2800, Ann Arbor, MI 48109-2800, USA; [c] Department of Environmental Health Sciences, University of Michigan, 1415 Washington Heights, Ann Arbor, MI 48109-2029, USA
* Corresponding author. Division of Rheumatology, Department of Internal Medicine, University of Michigan Health System, North Campus Research Complex, B014 G236, 2800 Plymouth Road, SPC 2800, Ann Arbor, MI 48109-2800.
E-mail address: wmarder@med.umich.edu

Rheum Dis Clin N Am 43 (2017) 275–285
http://dx.doi.org/10.1016/j.rdc.2016.12.007
0889-857X/17/© 2017 Elsevier Inc. All rights reserved.

rheumatic.theclinics.com

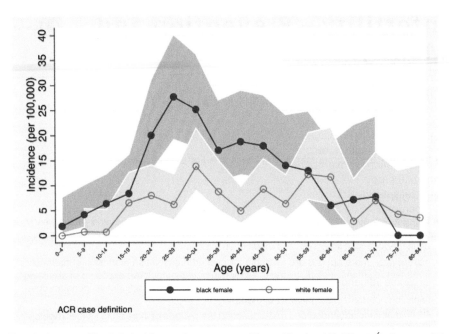

Fig. 1. Age-specific SLE incidence for women. (*From* Marder W, Vinet É, Somers EC. Rheumatic autoimmune diseases in women and midlife health. Women's Midlife Heal 2015;1(1):11.)

Underlying diminished ovarian reserve and lower parity rates have been observed in both rheumatic conditions and chronic diseases in general, and the use of alkylating agents for treatment of severe disease manifestations often causes ovarian damage. The increased recognition of broad health implications beyond fertility, related to ovarian damage, has heightened awareness of the need for ovarian protection during treatment with alkylating agents. In particular, the use of GnRH-a's during gonado-toxic therapy has become an acceptable option. A shift toward agents without gona-dotoxicity, such as mycophenolate mofetil and rituximab, has also reduced the risk of medication-related ovarian damage in rheumatic disease (RD) patients. This review summarizes current research and practice relating to rheumatic autoimmune diseases and fertility in women and outlines strategies for prevention of infertility. In men, auto-immune diseases, such as lupus, are rare and tend to have peak onset during late adulthood[4,5]; thus, the topic of infertility among male RD patients has not been thor-oughly investigated. Readers are referred, however, to a review elsewhere that covers male-specific considerations.[6]

PRIMARY OVARIAN INSUFFICIENCY

The term, *primary ovarian insufficiency (POI)*, is used when a woman less than 40 years old experiences amenorrhea for 4 months or more, with 2 serum follicle-stimulating hormone (FSH) levels obtained at least 1 month apart in the menopausal range.[7] POI is most frequently considered idiopathic, affecting 1% of women in the general population under the age of 40.[8] The term POI is preferred when discussing issues of subfertility, as opposed to terms, such as *primary ovarian failure* or *premature menopause*, because POI better reflects a continuum of impaired ovarian function rather than a dichotomous state.[9,10] This distinction is clinically important, because unlike natural menopause, which occurs at an average age of approximately 50 years, at least 50% of women with POI continue to experience variations in ovarian function, and anywhere between 5% and 10% conceive and deliver a child after a POI diagnosis.[11,12]

Antimüllerian hormone (AMH) is perhaps the most widely used and reliable serum biomarker of ovarian reserve and surrogate predictor for POI. AMH has demonstrated utility not only in predicting time to natural menopause, with serum levels declining to very low and nondetectable levels 5 years prior to the last menstrual period, but also for estimation of ovarian reserve in assisted reproductive therapy (ART) and after chemotherapy.[13–15] AMH is produced in the granulosa cells of the ovarian follicles and reflects the transition of resting primordial follicles into growing follicles. The ovarian pool of oocytes and their reproductive potential decline with age, and such decline is accelerated by exposure to chemotherapeutic agents. AMH is more highly correlated with the antral follicle count than are other reproductive hormones, such as FSH, luteinizing hormone, and estradiol.[16] AMH, furthermore, varies less across the menstrual cycle compared with other biomarkers of ovarian activity and does not seem to be influenced by chronic underlying disease, making it an excellent biomarker for studies of ovarian function in women with RD.[17–19]

In the absence of treatment with alkylating agents, some studies have observed no differences in POI prevalence between women with rheumatic autoimmune diseases and normal populations.[20–22] These studies, however, have focused primarily on menstrual histories and cessation of menses as outcomes and not on biologic markers of ovarian reserve. Other studies examining AMH levels reveal mixed results: studies of women with RDs, including SLE, rheumatoid arthritis, spondyloarthropathy, Takayasu arteritis, and Behçet syndrome, without prior exposure to cytotoxic medications found significantly diminished levels of AMH among women with these diseases compared with age-matched healthy controls.[23–27] No correlation was observed between disease activity measures and AMH levels, although disease activity in these studies was generally mild.

What is unknown, however, is the extent to which depressed markers of ovarian reserve in these patients represents the long-term effects of systemic inflammatory disease and the underlying mechanisms. Conversely, a case-control study of 80 premenopausal women with SLE and age-matched controls revealed no differences in AMH levels between groups and no associations between lupus disease activity or disease duration and AMH.[28]

ALTERATIONS IN THE HYPOTHALAMIC-PITUITARY-GONADAL AXIS

Studies of women with rheumatic autoimmune diseases, primarily SLE, have revealed alterations in the functioning of the HPG axis as well as menstrual irregularities. In a study of 30 juvenile SLE (JSLE) patients, the mean age of menarche was significantly older in JSLE than controls (13.1 years vs 11.6 years), and significantly more menstrual disturbances (including higher FSH and lower progesterone and luteinizing hormone levels) and longer length cycles were also observed.[29] There was no significant difference in the rate of menstrual irregularities between JSLE patients who had previously received CYC and those who had not. Although these findings support the possibility of HPG axis dysfunction and diminished ovarian reserve, AMH levels, arguably a more accurate assessment of ovarian reserve, were not assessed. Another study of 298 female JSLE patients receiving CYC revealed amenorrhea in 11.7% and normal FSH and estradiol levels for their ages. The CYC exposure was comparable in patients with and without amenorrhea; however, lupus diseases activity indices were significantly higher among those with amenorrhea, suggesting the possibility that disease activity and not HPG axis leads to menstrual irregularities in these patients.[30]

PARITY IN WOMEN WITH AUTOIMMUNE DISEASES

Prior to advances in therapies and disease management, many women with RDs were discouraged from having children for multiple reasons, including concerns that disease flare during pregnancy could affect their health or their baby's health and that disease-related disability might have an impact on their ability to care for a child.[31] This widely held sentiment is reflected in part in observed rates of decreased parity and smaller family size among women with SLE and different types of inflammatory arthritis.[32–35] A 2012 study of 852 women with rheumatoid arthritis (RA) and 165 women with SLE found that more than half of those who received their diagnoses prior to completing childbearing had fewer children than they had originally planned.[34] Underlying factors cited by the subjects included infertility rates among women with RA, pregnancy loss among women with SLE, and, in both groups, concerns that their disease would have an adverse impact on their offspring as well as family life. Supporting these observations is a large body of work describing concerns related to pregnancy and childcare that are common to many women with chronic diseases and are well documented among women with inflammatory arthritis. Survey studies have revealed that issues surrounding family planning have a significant impact on women with RDs, including disease-related physical limitations, balancing antenatal medication exposure and disease control, and uncertainty about the physical, social, and psychological challenges that come with motherhood, all of which can lead to significant anxiety surrounding reproductive choices.[3,36–39]

Ultimately, these concerns may manifest in choices made by women with RA to have fewer children than they had planned or remain childless altogether.[37,40] A large Norwegian study found a higher proportion of women with chronic inflammatory arthritis (including RA and idiopathic juvenile arthritis) treated with disease-modifying antirheumatic medications (DMARDs) or biologic agents were nulliparous compared with a randomly selected age-matched reference population: 32.6% of inflammatory arthritis patients were nulliparous versus 26.4% in reference population ($P<.001$).[32] Furthermore, although adjusted relative fertility rates in patients with chronic inflammatory arthritis before their diagnoses were not reduced, after diagnosis, the relative fertility rates were significantly lower in these populations.

A prolonged time to pregnancy (TTP) has also been observed among patients with RA prior to conception.[41,42] In a Dutch cohort of pregnant women with RA, 42% of the patients had a TTP exceeding 12 months, significantly longer than TTP among women in a comparable general Western European population, in which 50% of women have a TTP of 3 months and approximately 70% have TTP of 6 months after starting unprotected intercourse.[43] Age, nulliparity, disease activity, and preconception use of nonsteroidal anti-inflammatory drugs and dose-dependent prednisone therapy (significantly longer if >7.5 mg) were all independently associated with TTP. Autoantibodies, past DMARD use, smoking, and disease duration did not affect TTP.

Encouragingly, a recent study of national health care databases has revealed an increase in the numbers of children born to mothers with inflammatory arthritis. A 2016 study looked at trends in birth rates over time among women in Norway with inflammatory joint disease and found higher parity rates, particularly from 1990s onward[44];

this trend may in part reflect the development of better and safer treatment options, in particular the use of anti–tumor necrosis factor agents in the 1990s.

EFFECTS OF MEDICATIONS ON OVARIAN FUNCTION
Alkylating Agents

CYC and chlorambucil have been widely used in the treatment of severe autoimmune disease, in particular lupus nephritis.[45] Although chlorambucil is used less frequently, CYC continues to have an important role for treating severe organ-threatening manifestations of systemic autoimmune diseases, although increasingly less so, because studies support the use of mycophenolate mofetil and lower dose Euro-Lupus CYC regimens for induction of remission in proliferative lupus nephritis,[46–49] and rituximab for use in antineutrophil cytoplasmic antibody–associated vasculitis.[50]

CYC-induced ovarian toxicities reported in animal models include DNA cross-linking of granulosa cells, reduced numbers of granulosa cells, ovarian fibrosis, and decreased progesterone and estrogen.[51,52] In humans, CYC has been shown to impair follicle maturation and is associated with a dose-dependent depletion of the primordial antral follicle pool.[53] In lupus, CYC-associated premature ovarian failure occurs in 16% to 54% of patients[54–57] and is strongly associated with age at CYC initiation and cumulative dose.[56,58] Gradations of ovarian insult have also been observed: among women (mean age 35 years) with granulomatosis with polyangiitis in a trial of daily oral CYC or methotrexate, AMH levels declined by 0.74 ng/mL for each 10 g of CYC, highlighting the impact of oral CYC even for courses of less than 6 months.[59]

PRESERVATION OF FERTILITY IN WOMEN RECEIVING GONADOTOXIC THERAPIES
Assisted Reproductive Technologies

Women facing the prospect of gonadotoxic therapies should have the opportunity to discuss their options with a reproductive endocrinologist. Although embryo cryopreservation is a proved ART method, the requirements for an available partner/sperm and several weeks of preparation limit its utility in patients facing treatment of cancer or severe manifestations of autoimmune disease.[60] The 2013 guidelines issued by the Society for Reproductive Medicine and Society for Assisted Reproductive Technology state that given dramatic improvements in the success of oocyte cryopreservation, this technique should no longer be considered experimental and should be recommended, with appropriate counseling, in patients at risk of infertility due to chemotherapy or gonadotoxic therapies.[61]

There is no evidence that fertility success rates or the number of in vitro fertilization (IVF) cycles among women with RDs undergoing ART differ from the general population; however, studies have suggested worse outcomes if disease is active in pregnancy.[62–65] Antiphospholipid antibody positivity also does not seem to influence IVF outcomes.[66] Hormonal manipulations specific to particular ART strategies, however, and potential implications related to estrogen levels, disease flare, or thrombosis should be evaluated in the context of the individual patient's underlying disease and risk factors.[6]

Procedures involving ART generally require planning, for example, 12 days are allowed for maturation of oocytes prior to retrieval, so they are less attractive if treatment with CYC is indicated urgently. Both procedures are associated with medication costs of controlled ovarian hyperstimulation, retrieval costs, thawing and transfer costs, and yearly storage fees that can run into tens of thousands of dollars.

Experimental ART methods, such as ovarian tissue cryopreservation, may also warrant exploration in the patient population exposed to gonadotoxic drugs.

Gonadotropin-releasing Hormone Analog Therapy

Given the numerous health concerns associated with POI, including increased risk of cardiovascular disease, bone loss, mental health comorbidities, and all-cause mortality,[67] mitigation of ovarian damage associated with gonadotoxic therapy should be a treatment goal even among women who do not desire future pregnancy. Temporary ovarian suppression with GnRH-a therapy concurrent with chemotherapy administration is a promising strategy for ovarian protection. Although still considered investigational, it is attractive due to its noninvasive nature and potential to provide protection against ovarian damage and forestall premature ovarian insufficiency. Aside from treatment regimens designed to limit cumulative exposure to gonadotoxic drugs (eg, Euro-Lupus regimen[48]), adjunctive GnRH-a therapy currently is the most promising strategy available for ovarian preservation rather than solely maintenance of reproductive capacity. It is also less costly and invasive than other ART procedures.

GnRH-a for ovarian preservation has been examined in both cancer and autoimmune populations undergoing various chemotherapeutic regimens. The authors' group was among the first to report a benefit of GnRH-a for protection against premature ovarian failure among women with severe lupus on a standard CYC regimen.[68] As shown by the time-to-event analysis in **Fig. 2**, cumulative preservation of ovarian function after CYC therapy was significantly greater among women treated with adjunctive GnRH-a compared with controls matched by age and cumulative CYC dose. The endpoint of premature ovarian failure in this study was defined as

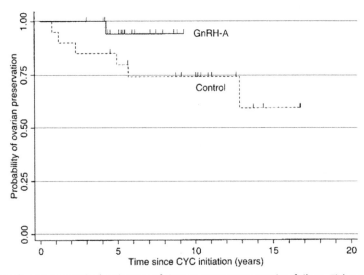

Fig. 2. Kaplan-Meier survival estimates of time to premature ovarian failure. Tick marks indicate censored observations (ie, the final point of follow-up for patients who did not develop the endpoint of premature ovarian failure). (*From* Somers EC, Marder W, Christman GM, et al. Use of a gonadotropin-releasing hormone analog for protection against premature ovarian failure during cyclophosphamide therapy in women with severe lupus. Arthritis Rheum 2005;52:2763; with permission.)

amenorrhea of at least 12 months' duration and an FSH level greater than or equal to 40 mIU/mL.

GnRH-a may also provide gradations of benefit for ovarian health, as measured by biomarkers of ovarian function. The authors found higher post-CYC levels of AMH among women who received adjunctive GnRH-a during CYC therapy.[69] A review published in 2015 found that on aggregate GnRH-a was positively associated with benefit based on 20 studies inclusive of 2038 patients; benefit was not detected in 8 studies inclusive of 509 patients.[70]

The standard GnRH-a protocol is comprised of 3.75-mg depot leuprolide acetate (a GnRH agonist) injection once per month throughout CYC therapy.[68] To reduce ovarian CYC exposure during the initial estrogen surge associated with GnRH-a, the injection is ideally timed to precede the subsequent monthly intravenous CYC bolus by approximately 10 days to 14 days. For CYC courses started on an urgent basis, initiation of GnRH-a is generally postponed until after the first monthly intravenous CYC (although exception to this may be contemplated for women in the luteal phase of their menstrual cycle, when an estrogen flare is less likely). In the clinical setting, patients tolerating the first 30-day GnRH-a dose may subsequently be switched to quarterly injection. To reduce symptoms of hormone withdrawal, transdermal estrogen may be considered, if not otherwise contraindicated (eg, a hypercoagulable state, such as antiphospholipid antibody syndrome), to maintain slightly less than physiologic estrogen (early follicular phase) levels.

The various strategies for preserving fertility, discussed previously, are not mutually exclusive, and often multiple options may be integrated in an effort to optimize outcomes. Close collaboration with reproductive endocrinology specialists is essential to design an individualized plan taking into account patient goals and preferences.

SUMMARY

Infertility and subfertility, menstrual irregularities, and decreased parity may occur in women with autoimmune diseases due to multiple factors, including underlying inflammatory disease, gonadotoxic medications, and psychosocial issues related to living with chronic disease. Awareness of these factors, as well as validation and support of patients confronting reproductive challenges, is important for providing comprehensive care to these women. In particular, an understanding of the expanding options for fertility preservation strategies during gonadotoxic medications is essential, including GnRH-a cotherapy and oocyte cryopreservation. Referral to a reproductive endocrinology clinic is indicated in this patient population, in part to help manage symptoms of hypoestrogenism that may result from GnRH-a therapy.

REFERENCES

1. Cooper GS, Bynum MLK, Somers EC. Recent insights in the epidemiology of autoimmune diseases: improved prevalence estimates and understanding of clustering of diseases. J Autoimmun 2009;33(3–4):197–207.

2. Somers EC, Marder W, Cagnoli P, et al. Population-based incidence and prevalence of systemic lupus erythematosus: the Michigan lupus epidemiology and surveillance program. Arthritis Rheumatol 2014;66(2):369–78.

3. Marder W, Vinet É, Somers EC. Rheumatic autoimmune diseases in women and midlife health. Women's Midlife Heal 2015;1(1):11.

4. Cooper GS, Stroehla BC. The epidemiology of autoimmune diseases. Autoimmun Rev 2003;2(3):119–25.

5. Somers EC, Thomas SL, Smeeth L, et al. Incidence of systemic lupus erythematosus in the United Kingdom, 1990-1999. Arthritis Rheum 2007;57(4):612–8.
6. Hickman RA, Gordon C. Causes and management of infertility in systemic lupus erythematosus. Rheumatology (Oxford) 2011;50(9):1551–8.
7. Nelson LM. Clinical practice. Primary ovarian insufficiency. N Engl J Med 2009; 360(6):606–14.
8. Coulam CB, Adamson SC, Annegers JF. Incidence of premature ovarian failure. Obstet Gynecol 1986;67(4):604–6.
9. Welt CK. Primary ovarian insufficiency: a more accurate term for premature ovarian failure. Clin Endocrinol (Oxf) 2008;68(4):499–509.
10. Kalantaridou SN, Nelson LM. Premature ovarian failure is not premature menopause. Ann N Y Acad Sci 2000;900:393–402.
11. van Noord PA, Dubas JS, Dorland M, et al. Age at natural menopause in a population-based screening cohort: the role of menarche, fecundity, and lifestyle factors. Fertil Steril 1997;68(1):95–102.
12. Rebar RW. Premature ovarian failure. Obstet Gynecol 2009;113(6):1355–63.
13. Majumder K, Gelbaya TA, Laing I, et al. The use of anti-Müllerian hormone and antral follicle count to predict the potential of oocytes and embryos. Eur J Obstet Gynecol Reprod Biol 2010;150(2):166–70.
14. Sowers MR, Eyvazzadeh AD, McConnell D, et al. Anti-mullerian hormone and inhibin B in the definition of ovarian aging and the menopause transition. J Clin Endocrinol Metab 2008;93(9):3478–83.
15. Visser JA, Schipper I, Laven JSE, et al. Anti-Müllerian hormone: an ovarian reserve marker in primary ovarian insufficiency. Nat Rev Endocrinol 2012;8(6): 331–41.
16. Fanchin R, Schonäuer LM, Righini C, et al. Serum anti-Müllerian hormone is more strongly related to ovarian follicular status than serum inhibin B, estradiol, FSH and LH on day 3. Hum Reprod 2003;18(2):323–7.
17. La Marca A, Grisendi V, Griesinger G. How much does AMH really vary in normal women? Int J Endocrinol 2013;2013:1–8.
18. La Marca A, Sighinolfi G, Radi D, et al. Anti-Mullerian hormone (AMH) as a predictive marker in assisted reproductive technology (ART). Hum Reprod Update 2011;16(2):113–30.
19. Visser JA, de Jong FH, Laven JS, et al. Anti-Müllerian hormone: a new marker for ovarian function. Reproduction 2006;131(1):1–9.
20. Pasoto SG, Mendonça BB, Bonfá E. Menstrual disturbances in patients with systemic lupus erythematosus without alkylating therapy: clinical, hormonal and therapeutic associations. Lupus 2002;11(3):175–80.
21. Alpízar-Rodríguez D, Romero-Díaz J, Sánchez-Guerrero J, et al. Age at natural menopause among patients with systemic lupus erythematosus. Rheumatology (Oxford) 2014;53(11):2023–9.
22. Mayorga J, Alpízar-Rodríguez D, Prieto-Padilla J, et al. Prevalence of premature ovarian failure in patients with systemic lupus erythematosus. Lupus 2016;25: 675–83.
23. Henes M, Froeschlin J, Taran FA, et al. Ovarian reserve alterations in premenopausal women with chronic inflammatory rheumatic diseases: impact of rheumatoid arthritis, Behçet's disease and spondyloarthritis on anti-Müllerian hormone levels. Rheumatology (Oxford) 2015;54(9):1709–12.
24. Wei W, Lin Q, Huang Q, et al. Impact of systemic lupus erythematosus on ovarian reserve in premenopausal women before receiving cyclophosphamide therapy: evaluation using anti-Müllerian hormone. Adv Reprod Sci 2016;04(01):17–22.

25. Yamakami LYS, Serafini PC, de Araujo DB, et al. Ovarian reserve in women with primary antiphospholipid syndrome. Lupus 2014;23(9):862–7.
26. Mont'Alverne ARS, Pereira RMR, Yamakami LYS, et al. Reduced ovarian reserve in patients with Takayasu arteritis. J Rheumatol 2014;41(10):2055–9.
27. Lawrenz B, Henes J, Henes M, et al. Impact of systemic lupus erythematosus on ovarian reserve in premenopausal women: evaluation by using anti-Muellerian hormone. Lupus 2011;20(11):1193–7.
28. Gasparin AA, Souza L, Siebert M, et al. Assessment of anti-Müllerian hormone levels in premenopausal patients with systemic lupus erythematosus. Lupus 2016;25(3):227–32.
29. Medeiros PB, Febrônio MV, Bonfá E, et al. Menstrual and hormonal alterations in juvenile systemic lupus erythematosus. Lupus 2009;18(1):38–43.
30. Silva CA, Yamakami LYS, Aikawa NE, et al. Autoimmune primary ovarian insufficiency. Autoimmun Rev 2014;13(4–5):427–30.
31. Ostensen M. Counselling women with rheumatic disease–how many children are desirable? Scand J Rheumatol 1991;20(2):121–6.
32. Wallenius M, Skomsvoll JF, Irgens LM, et al. Fertility in women with chronic inflammatory arthritides. Rheumatology 2011;50(6):1162–7.
33. Skomsvoll JF, Ostensen M, Baste V, et al. Number of births, interpregnancy interval, and subsequent pregnancy rate after a diagnosis of inflammatory rheumatic disease in Norwegian women. J Rheumatol 2001;28(10):2310–4.
34. Clowse MEB, Chakravarty E, Costenbader KH, et al. Effects of infertility, pregnancy loss, and patient concerns on family size of women with rheumatoid arthritis and systemic lupus erythematosus. Arthritis Care Res (Hoboken) 2012; 64(5):668–74.
35. Vinet E, Pineau C, Gordon C, et al. Systemic lupus erythematosus in women: Impact on family size. Arthritis Rheum 2008;59(11):1656–60.
36. Chakravarty EF. Rheumatoid arthritis and pregnancy: beyond smaller and preterm babies. Arthritis Rheum 2011;63(6):1469–71.
37. Katz PP. Childbearing decisions and family size among women with rheumatoid arthritis. Arthritis Rheum 2006;55(2):217–23.
38. Del Junco DJ, Annegers JF, Coulam CB, et al. The relationship between rheumatoid arthritis and reproductive function. Br J Rheumatol 1989;28(Suppl 1):33 [discussion: 42–5].
39. Meade T, Sharpe L, Hallab L, et al. Navigating motherhood choices in the context of rheumatoid arthritis: women's stories. Musculoskeletal Care 2013;11(2):73–82.
40. Ostensen M. Pregnancy in patients with a history of juvenile rheumatoid arthritis. Arthritis Rheum 1991;34(7):881–7.
41. Jawaheer D, Zhu JL, Nohr EA, et al. Time to pregnancy among women with rheumatoid arthritis. Arthritis Rheum 2011;63(6):1517–21.
42. Brouwer J, Hazes JMW, Laven JSE, et al. Fertility in women with rheumatoid arthritis: influence of disease activity and medication. Ann Rheum Dis 2015; 74(10):1836–41.
43. Juul S, Karmaus W, Olsen J. Regional differences in waiting time to pregnancy: pregnancy-based surveys from Denmark, France, Germany, Italy and Sweden. The European Infertility and Subfecundity Study Group. Hum Reprod 1999; 14(5):1250–4.
44. Wallenius M, Salvesen KÅ, Daltveit AK, et al. Reproductive trends in females with inflammatory joint disease. BMC Pregnancy Childbirth 2016;16(1):123.
45. Marder W, McCune WJ. Advances in immunosuppressive therapy. Semin Respir Crit Care Med 2007;28(4):398–417.

46. Ginzler EM, Dooley MA, Aranow C, et al. Mycophenolate mofetil or intravenous cyclophosphamide for lupus nephritis. N Engl J Med 2005;353(21):2219–28.
47. Appel GB, Contreras G, Dooley MA, et al. Mycophenolate mofetil versus cyclophosphamide for induction treatment of lupus nephritis. J Am Soc Nephrol 2009;20(5):1103–12.
48. Houssiau FA, Vasconcelos C, D'Cruz D, et al. Immunosuppressive therapy in lupus nephritis: the Euro-Lupus Nephritis Trial, a randomized trial of low-dose versus high-dose intravenous cyclophosphamide. Arthritis Rheum 2002;46(8): 2121–31.
49. Houssiau FA, Vasconcelos C, D'Cruz D, et al. The 10-year follow-up data of the Euro-Lupus Nephritis Trial comparing low-dose and high-dose intravenous cyclophosphamide. Ann Rheum Dis 2010;69(1):61–4.
50. Stone JH, Merkel PA, Spiera R, et al. Rituximab versus Cyclophosphamide for ANCA-Associated Vasculitis. N Engl J Med 2010;363(3):221–32.
51. Slater CA, Liang MH, McCune JW, et al. Preserving ovarian function in patients receiving cyclophosphamide. Lupus 1999;8(1):3–10.
52. Ataya KM, Valeriote FA, Ramahi-Ataya AJ. Effect of cyclophosphamide on the immature rat ovary. Cancer Res 1989;49(7):1660–4.
53. Warne GL, Fairley KF, Hobbs JB, et al. Cyclophosphamide-induced ovarian failure. N Engl J Med 1973;289(22):1159–62.
54. Clowse MEB, Behera MA, Anders CK, et al. Ovarian preservation by GnRH Agonists during chemotherapy: a meta-analysis. J Womens Health 2009;18(3): 311–9.
55. Park M-C, Park Y-B, Jung SY, et al. Risk of ovarian failure and pregnancy outcome in patients with lupus nephritis treated with intravenous cyclophosphamide pulse therapy. Lupus 2004;13(8):569–74.
56. McDermott EM, Powell RJ. Incidence of ovarian failure in systemic lupus erythematosus after treatment with pulse cyclophosphamide. Ann Rheum Dis 1996; 55(4):224–9.
57. Boumpas DT, Austin HA 3rd, Vaughan EM, et al. Risk for sustained amenorrhea in patients with systemic lupus erythematosus receiving intermittent pulse cyclophosphamide therapy. Ann Intern Med 1993;119(5):366–9.
58. Mok CC, Lau CS, Wong RW. Risk factors for ovarian failure in patients with systemic lupus erythematosus receiving cyclophosphamide therapy. Arthritis Rheum 1998;41(5):831–7.
59. Clowse MEB, Copland SC, Hsieh T-C, et al. Ovarian reserve diminished by oral cyclophosphamide therapy for granulomatosis with polyangiitis (Wegener's). Arthritis Care Res (Hoboken) 2011;63(12):1777–81.
60. ASRM/ART PC. Ovarian tissue and oocyte cryopreservation. Fertil Steril 2004; 82(4):993–8.
61. ASRM/ART PC. Mature oocyte cryopreservation: a guideline. Fertil Steril 2013; 99(1):37–43.
62. Guballa N, Sammaritano L, Schwartzman S, et al. Ovulation induction and in vitro fertilization in systemic lupus erythematosus and antiphospholipid syndrome. Arthritis Rheum 2000;43(3):550–6.
63. Di Nisio M, Rutjes AWS, Ferrante N, et al. Thrombophilia and outcomes of assisted reproduction technologies: a systematic review and meta-analysis. Blood 2011;118(10):2670–8.
64. Steinvil A, Raz R, Berliner S, et al. Association of common thrombophilias and antiphospholipid antibodies with success rate of in vitro fertilisation. Thromb Haemost 2012;108(6):1192–7.

65. Levine AB, Lockshin MD. Assisted reproductive technology in SLE and APS. Lupus 2014;23(12):1239–41.
66. Chighizola CB, de Jesus GR. Antiphospholipid antibodies and infertility. Lupus 2014;23(12):1232–8.
67. Marder W, Fisseha S, Ganser MA, et al. Ovarian damage during chemotherapy in autoimmune diseases: broad health implications beyond fertility. Clin Med Insights Reprod Health 2012;2012(6):9–18.
68. Somers EC, Marder W, Christman GM, et al. Use of a gonadotropin-releasing hormone analog for protection against premature ovarian failure during cyclophosphamide therapy in women with severe lupus. Arthritis Rheum 2005;52:2761–7.
69. Marder W, McCune WJ, Wang L, et al. Adjunctive GnRH-a treatment attenuates depletion of ovarian reserve associated with cyclophosphamide therapy in premenopausal SLE patients. Gynecol Endocrinol 2012;28(8):624–7.
70. Blumenfeld Z, Evron A. Preserving fertility when choosing chemotherapy regimens - the role of gonadotropin-releasing hormone agonists. Expert Opin Pharmacother 2015;16(7):1009–20.

Menopause and Rheumatic Disease

Mitali Talsania, MBBS[a], Robert Hal Scofield, MD[a,b,c],*

KEYWORDS

- Menopause • Systemic lupus erythematosus • Osteoarthritis • Rheumatoid arthritis

KEY POINTS

- Menopause, and its treatment, may affect rheumatic diseases; rheumatic diseases may affect menopause.
- Treatment with cyclophosphamide, especially at an older age, may induce menopause.
- Decreased ovarian reserve is a feature intrinsic to disease notwithstanding treatment.
- Osteoporosis is common in several rheumatic diseases, and menopause increases the risk of osteoporosis as well as fragility fracture.
- The effect of menopause and its treatment is difficult to define in osteoarthritis because of contradictory results.

INTRODUCTION

Menopause is defined as cessation of menses retrospectively for 12 months without a pathophysiologic cause. However, age-related changes in ovarian function begin in the middle of the fourth decade of life with decreased ovarian follicles. Resultant changes in hypothalamic and pituitary hormones to compensate for the falling reserve of ovarian follicles maintain ovulation and fertility, sometimes for decades. The transition to the menopausal state demonstrates highly variable cyclic follicle development and ovulation, along with disrupted menstrual bleeding patterns.[1] The average age at menopause is about 51 years with later age of menopause correlating with longevity.[2–15]

Rheumatic illnesses include diseases with evidence of autoimmunity as well as the common, near ubiquitous, osteoarthritis (OA). These diseases are generally more common among women compared with men. There are extensive data describing

Disclosures: The authors have nothing to disclose.
[a] Section of Endocrinology, Diabetes and Metabolism, Department of Medicine, College of Medicine, University of Oklahoma Health Sciences Center, 1000 Lincoln Blvd, Oklahoma City, OK 73104, USA; [b] Arthritis & Clinical Immunology Program, Oklahoma Medical Research Foundation, 825 Northeast 13th Street, MS 24, Oklahoma City, OK 73104, USA; [c] Medical Service, Department of Veterans Affairs Medical Center, 920 NE 13th Street, Oklahoma City, OK 73104, USA
* Corresponding author. 825 Northeast 13th Street, MS 24, Oklahoma City, OK 73104.
E-mail address: hal-scofield@omrf.ouhsc.edu

Rheum Dis Clin N Am 43 (2017) 287–302
http://dx.doi.org/10.1016/j.rdc.2016.12.011
0889-857X/17/Published by Elsevier Inc.

rheumatic.theclinics.com

the relationship of some diseases with the menopausal state, whereas the data are scant for other rheumatic diseases. In this review, the authors consider the impact of menopause on several of these diseases and the reverse, that is, the impact of the diseases on menopause.

SYSTEMIC LUPUS ERYTHEMATOSUS

Systemic lupus erythematosus (SLE) is the prototype systemic inflammatory rheumatic disease. There is a wide range of serologic and clinical manifestations attributed to SLE with virtually every patient having a unique disease course. The disease affects women about 10 times more commonly than men with onset typically in the third or fourth decade of life.[16] Despite the usual onset well before the average age of menopause, there is a wealth of data concerning menopause and SLE, with multiple aspects of this relationship to consider. Among these are whether age of onset of menopause is a risk factor for SLE and whether onset of menopause alters the course or severity of the disease or its complications, including accelerated cardiovascular disease. Hormonal therapy for menopause may also interact with the disease. Disease with onset after menopause, although uncommon, may be a distinct entity compared with premenopausal onset. Finally, cytotoxic therapy for SLE may induce an iatrogenic and early menopause. This review considers these aspects of SLE and menopause.

A recent cross-sectional study examined menopause in 961 patients with SLE, of whom 7.9% had natural menopause.[17] Meanwhile, 4.1% had undergone a hysterectomy and 6.3% had menopause after taking cyclophosphamide. Only a small number (0.1%) had menopause associated with end-stage renal disease. The mean age at menopause was 46.4 years and the median age was 50.7 years, both similar to reported values for the general population.[17] An early age at menopause was associated with an earlier age of SLE diagnosis, however.[17] In Lupus in Minorities: Nature versus Nurture (LUMINA) study, a multiethnic SLE cohort from the United States, 37 of 316 women had premature menopause. In a multivariable regression analysis, age at receiving cyclophosphamide, cyclophosphamide induction therapy, higher disease activity, and Texas-Hispanic heritage were associated with a premature gonadal failure.[18] Older studies also show age and cumulative dose of the drug as important predictors of premature menopause.[19] Another study compared prolonged intravenous (IV) cyclophosphamide with 5 to 7 monthly doses followed by mycophenolate mofetil. In the latter group only 1 of 22 women (4%) had sustained amenorrhea, whereas in patients with prolonged cyclophosphamide treatment, 20 of 39 (51%) had sustained amenorrhea. Once again, older age at initiation of treatment was an important risk factor.[20] Neutrophil count suppression by pulse IV cyclophosphamide[21] as well as hypothyroidism[22] may also predict premature ovarian failure. In the last study, 11 of 71 patients with SLE receiving cyclophosphamide developed ovarian failure: all 11 had hypothyroidism as evidenced by an elevated thyroid-stimulating hormone.[22] Thus, treatment with cyclophosphamide can induce premature menopause in women with SLE, especially when treatment begins at an older age (>32 years), whereas hypothyroidism as a risk factor is reported but not confirmed by subsequent studies.

Nonetheless, factors unrelated to cyclophosphamide can affect ovarian reserve in patients with SLE. Using levels of anti-Müllerian hormone (AMH) as a measure of ovarian function in a study of 33 premenopausal women with SLE (without past cyclophosphamide use) and 33 age- and ethnicity-matched healthy controls, Lawrenz and colleagues[23] found lower mean AMH in SLE (2.15 ± 1.64 vs 3.17 ± 2.29); however, there was no difference in number of pregnancies or spontaneous abortions between the groups. Another study confirmed this result but found AMH levels did not predict early menopause.[24] The factors intrinsic to SLE that affect ovarian function and reserve have not yet been identified. And, although antiovarian antibodies have been described in patients with SLE,[25] there is no evidence of premature menopause among patients with SLE apart from the effects of cyclophosphamide.[26] Pharmacologic suppression of ovarian function by gonadotropin-releasing hormone agonists may protect women from premature ovarian failure caused by this drug,[27,28] and there are several other strategies to preserve fertility after cyclophosphamide, including oocyte preservation.[29]

Whether or not menopause, natural or otherwise, affects the course of SLE has been investigated. This investigation includes the study of SLE with onset at an older, postmenopausal age. A study of SLE with average age of onset at 55 years among 20 postmenopausal and 70 premenopausal women showed the postmenopausal women were statistically less likely to have malar rash (55% vs 80%), renal disease (30% vs 69%), leukopenia (25% vs 56%), or positive antinuclear antibody (70% vs 93%).[30] Other studies find low incidence of anti–double-stranded DNA (dsDNA) and hypocomplementemia among postmenopausal SLE onset.[31] Thus, absence of these characteristic features, along with older age, may make diagnosis difficult.

Menopause may also affect the course of SLE. In a study of 34 postmenopausal patients with SLE with premenopausal onset compared with patients with SLE continuing to have menstrual periods, Mok and colleagues[32] found fewer (0.5/y vs 0.14/y) and less severe flares. Mean and maximum disease activity were both decreased in 30 patients with SLE not receiving sex hormone therapy followed for an average of 1.7 years before and 3.3 years after menopause.[33]

Surgical menopause before SLE onset was associated with less renal involvement and lower anti-dsDNA seropositivity, an effect independent of ethnicity.[34] However, the Toronto Lupus Group has shown a constant rate of improvement in disease activity over time since diagnosis regardless of onset of menopause, concluding that menopause is not a proximate cause of improved SLE disease activity.[35] That is, the evidence suggests that SLE improves after menopause but a cause and effect relationship has not been established.

The relationship of menopause to disease activity in SLE begs the controversial question of whether postmenopausal sex hormone replacement is safe in patients with SLE. This topic has been studied and reviewed extensively.[36,37] Evidence from the Nurses' Health Study, a large prospective cohort study, shows a 2-fold increased risk of SLE for women treated with postmenopausal hormone replacement.[38] However, these data were collected at a time when such therapy was much more common than now. Estrogen or combined estrogen-progesterone therapy[39] is associated with increased mild to moderate flares of SLE but not with severe flares.[37] New data are available that may suggest possible mechanisms of SLE flares with hormonal therapy. In a recent study of 35 patients with SLE and 15 controls, investigators found increased expression of toll-like receptor (TLR) 3, 7, and 9 on peripheral blood mononuclear cells when comparing patients with controls. Postmenopausal status among the patients was associated with a higher percentage of cells expressing TLRs.[40] Another study reported decreased tumor necrosis factor production by estrogen-treated peripheral blood mononuclear cells from patients with SLE.[41]

Menopause has been studied in relationship to complications of SLE, especially premature atherosclerosis and osteoporosis. Low bone density is associated with disease activity and damage accrual: osteoporosis is an intrinsic part of SLE that is not induced purely by treatment.[42] Menopause is a risk factor for more severe osteoporosis as well as fragility fracture. Postmenopausal patients with SLE were significantly more likely to have a vertebral compression fracture than premenopausal patients.[43]

Further, the 10-year risk of osteoporotic fracture is greater among women with SLE compared with matched controls, despite comparable bone mineral density values. This risk was predicted by premature menopause as well as cumulative glucocorticoid dose.[44] Treatment with either estrogen or selective estrogen agonists, such as raloxifene,[45] maintain bone density in postmenopausal patients with SLE. Newer data suggest that raloxifene does not worsen lupus flares, alter disease activity, or increase inflammatory markers in postmenopausal patients with SLE.[46] But the study is small (n = 62) and relatively short (12 months).[45]

Women with SLE have dramatically increased rates of cardiovascular disease such that, beginning about 10 years after diagnosis, this is the most common cause of death.[47] Interestingly, a correlate of premature cardiovascular disease, as measured by coronary artery calcification, is low bone mineral density.[48] There are several studies of vascular function, which may serve as a surrogate of vascular disease, in women with SLE. Pulse wave velocity measured at peripheral large arteries determines arterial elasticity. Postmenopausal patients with SLE (n = 96) had worsened pulse wave velocity compared with premenopausal patients (n = 124), but most of this difference was explained by age in a multivariate analysis. But higher cumulative organ damage and worsened renal function were associated with stiffer arteries in the postmenopausal group.[49] A more traditional measure of arterial function is flow-mediated dilatation, usually determined at the brachial artery. A meta-analysis of these studies found that although endothelium-dependent flow-mediated dilatation was impaired in patients with SLE, menopause was not an important determinate in multivariate analysis.[50,51]

RHEUMATOID ARTHRITIS

Rheumatoid arthritis (RA) affects about 1% of the worldwide population with a ratio of women to men of up to 6 to 1 in young adults,[52] but the sex ratio approaches 1 as age of onset increases.[53] The onset of disease is substantially older than that seen in SLE such that initial disease among women is common in postmenopausal years.[54] Extra-articular disease may rarely lead to life-threatening complications; but patients with RA have excess mortality from several causes, including cardiovascular, infectious, and hematological disease.[54] Similar to SLE and OA, there are multiple aspects of the disease potentially related to menopause.

First among these to consider is whether menopause increases the risk or severity of RA. In fact, the results of observational studies of both menopause and estrogenic hormones, either postmenopausal or contraception, are variable and discrepant.[55,56] A study from Belgium showed that first symptoms of RA had a mean time from onset of menopause of zero. The investigators suggested these data indicate that the average woman with RA has the onset of symptoms concurrent with menopause.[53] A recent study showed that menopause before 45 years of age (early menopause) was associated with milder RA.[57] Meanwhile, another study found early menopause was associated with postmenopausal onset of RA.[58–60] Thus, a definite conclusion about the effects of menopause on RA cannot be made.

Some observational studies, but not all, show hormone replacement therapy (HRT) or oral contraception improves disease among postmenopausal women.[56,61–69] Similar to cardiovascular disease risk of HRT, studies of RA risk may be confounded by the use of estrogen alone versus estrogen plus progesterone. A recent population-based epidemiologic study from Sweden showed a decreased risk of anti–cyclic citrullinated peptide-positive RA among postmenopausal women older than 50 years with most of this reduction occurring in women on combination HRT (odds ratio

0.3).[66] But in a 2-year study of HRT in 88 postmenopausal women with RA, there were no changes in autoantibodies.[70] In addition, a 6-month, randomized, single-blinded, placebo-controlled trial showed no improvement in RA.[71] But this last trial likely has no bearing on whether or not HRT reduces the risk of developing RA.

Similar to other inflammatory rheumatic illnesses, osteoporosis is caused in part by the disease itself with specific effects on bone remodeling and not simply a result of glucocorticoid therapy.[72] In a study of 343 postmenopausal and 100 premenopausal women with RA, 56% of the former but only 18% of the latter had osteoporosis.[73] Of course, study of healthy women before and after menopause might find similar numbers. However, there is clearly excess osteoporosis among women with RA compared with controls with postmenopausal status an important predictor.[74] Excess bone loss seen in RA occurs early in the disease.[75] Recent studies from the era of biologics (and low prevalence of postmenopausal HRT) continue to show excess osteoporosis in patients with RA compared with age-matched controls (30.0% vs 17.4%) and an association with menopause.[76] HRT reduces bone resorption regardless of glucocorticoid therapy in postmenopausal patients with RA[77–85]; but there are, of course, other potential health concerns with postmenopausal HRT.

OSTEOARTHRITIS

OA is highly prevalent in postmenopausal women. The Women's Health Initiative showed that 44% of the participating postmenopausal women reported OA. Risk factors in this study include higher body mass index and older age. American Indian and African American women in the extreme obesity category have significant odds of OA compared with non-Hispanic white women.[86–91]

Estrogen receptors are present in joint tissues. Estrogen has chondro-protective roles in part due to glycosaminoglycan synthesis, which is an important part of connective tissue. Estrogen also inhibits cyclooxygenase 2 messenger RNA expression in bovine articular chondrocytes as well as other tissues, leading to protection against reactive oxygen species induced chondrocyte damage.[92] Estrogens decrease cartilage damage. Coincubation of chondrocytes with interleukin (IL)-1b and raloxifene led to a dose-dependent increase in proteoglycans and reduction of matrix metalloproteinase-3 and nitric oxide induced by IL-1b.[93] Polymorphism in the estrogen receptor (ER) alpha gene may be associated with risk of severe OA of large, lower limb joints in a sex-specific manner suggesting that estrogen activity may influence the development of large joint OA.[94] The same study concluded that variation in aromatase gene CYP19A1 and ER alpha gene is associated with risk of severe OA. Influence of the CYP19A1 single nucleotide polymorphism is more important in women than in men and in knee OA than in hip OA.[94] A recent meta-analysis by Ma and colleagues[95] reported rs9340799 and rs2228480 polymorphisms, rather than the rs2234693 polymorphism, in the ER alpha gene are associated with the incidence of OA.

It has been demonstrated that C-telopeptide of type II collagen (CTX II), a marker of collagen degradation, increases in the urine of asymptomatic postmenopausal women and ovariectomized rats, suggesting that estrogen deprivation leads to cartilage breakdown. No association has been found for urinary Helix II and estrogen deprivation leading to cartilage breakdown.[96] A study of 860 women in China noted that menopause is associated with cartilage degeneration of the knee joint compared with premenopausal and perimenopausal women. Knee cartilage showed progressive severe degeneration on MRI in the first 2.5 years since menopause. However, although the investigators reported controlling for age, the study did not achieve much overlap in age across the menopause status group. The investigators concluded that estrogen deficiency is a risk factor for cartilage degeneration, and further studies are needed to clarify whether age or menopause plays a more important role in progression of cartilage degeneration.[97–99] The study could not definitely differentiate between the effects of menopause and age in our opinion.

Gao and colleagues studied endogenous estrogens and estrogen metabolites in premenopausal and postmenopausal Chinese women with OA.[100] The study showed that serum concentration of free estradiol and total 2-hydroxyestrone were significantly lower in premenopausal women with OA compared with the levels in controls (RA and healthy women). In postmenopausal women, serum concentration of free and total estradiol was significantly decreased compared with controls, and 2-hydroxyestradiol was significantly increased in postmenopausal women.[101] The investigators reported that apart from free and total estradiol deficiency, a decreased serum level of total 2-hydroxyestrone in premenopausal women and an increased total 2-hydroxyestradiol level in postmenopausal women with OA may correlate with the pathogenesis of OA.[100,101]

Studies on hormonal therapy in postmenopausal women with OA have shown conflicting evidence (**Table 1**). The Women's Health Initiative study showed that there are 29% greater odds of OA with past HRT use and 38% greater odds of OA for current HRT. American Indian women who reported current HRT use had an odds ratio of greater than 2 for arthritis (presumably OA) than the population as a whole.[86] In contrast, an Italian study showed HRT is associated with 27% lower odds ratio of physician-diagnosed OA.[102] In a cohort study of 1001 postmenopausal women (mean age 71 years) the effect of postmenopausal estrogen therapy was examined on hand, knee, and hip OA. A total of 638 women had used estrogen after menopause for greater than 1 year, and 71% were current users. Postmenopausal estrogen use for greater than 1 year was associated with higher prevalence of OA compared with no use of estrogen (34.5% compared with 30.9%, $P = .02$). Women using estrogen had significantly higher prevalence of hip and hand OA (15.8% vs 13.5%, $P = .02$ for hip, 4.1% compared with 1.1%, $P = .002$ for hand). Knee OA was slightly higher with estrogen use; however, the difference was not statistically significant. Unfortunately, this study did not report radiographic evidence of OA.[103] In contrast, a large cross-sectional study evaluated 4366 postmenopausal women for osteoporotic fractures. Women currently using estrogen had 40% lower prevalence of radiologic and symptomatic hip OA. Reduction was greater for estrogen use greater than 10 years.[104] In the Framingham OA study, estrogen use was not associated with increased risk of radiographic OA of the knees. In fact, estrogen use had a modest but nonsignificant protective effect in the study.[105] In the Heart and Estrogen/Progestin Replacement Study, older postmenopausal women with cardiac disease (n = 969) were assessed for knee pain. There was no significant effect of 4 years of estrogen plus progestin therapy compared with placebo on knee pain and related disability, indicating that HRT is not associated with more prevalent or severe knee pain.[106] The Chingford cross-sectional study demonstrated an inverse association of current postmenopausal HRT use and radiologic knee OA, suggesting protective effects. There was a nonsignificant protective effect for distal interphalangeal OA but no clear effect on carpometacarpal joints, leading to the conclusion that the effect was weaker in the hand joints.[107] Further studies are needed to evaluate the true effect of estrogen replacement on OA considering the current contradictory evidence. Consideration of the site of OA may be critical in any such study.

The effect of hormone therapy on risk of hip and knee joint replacement was evaluated in the Women's Health Initiative study. The population included postmenopausal women aged 50 to 79 years who were followed for a mean of 7.1 years. Women

Table 1
Effect of postmenopausal hormone replacement on osteoarthritis

Study	Type of Study	Population	Results
Women's Health Initiative[86]	Observational study	N = 146,494 Postmenopausal women	• HRT use associated with increased odds of OA • 29% increase odds of OA with current use and 38% with past use of HRT
Parazzini & Progretto Menopausa Italia Study Group,[102] 2003	Cross-sectional study	N = 42,464 Italian postmenopausal women	• Increase odds of OA with menopause • Natural menopause associated with increased OR of 1.13 for OA (95% CI 1.07, 1.21) • Surgical menopause OR of 1.18 for OA (95% CI 1.09, 1.28) • HRT: 27% lower odds of physician-diagnosed OA compared with those not on HRT
Von Mühlen et al,[103] 2002	Cross-sectional study	N = 1001 Postmenopausal women	• Postmenopausal estrogen use: 34% higher prevalence of OA compared with nonusers • Higher prevalence of subjects with hip and hand OA using estrogen replacement therapy compared with nonusers (15.8% compared with 13.5%, $P = .02$ for hip, 4.1% compared with 1.1%, $P = .002$ for hand)
Nevitt et al,[104] 1996	Cross-sectional study	N = 4366 Postmenopausal women	• 40% Lower prevalence for radiologic and symptomatic OA of hip with estrogen use
Framingham OA Study[105]	Cohort study	N = 831	• Nonsignificant protective effect for radiographic knee OA (OR 0.71, 95% CI 0.42, 1.20) or severe radiographic OA (OR 0.66, 95% CI 0.33, 1.32) with estrogen use
Heart Estrogen/Progestin Replacement Study[106]	Randomized control trial	N = 969 Postmenopausal women	• No difference between women on HRT vs placebo on knee pain and related disability
Chingford Study[107]	Cross-sectional study	N = 606 Postmenopausal women	• Current HRT use was protective for knee OA (OR 0.31, 95% CI 0.11, 0.93) • Nonsignificant protective effect for OA of DIP joint with HRT use; OR 0.48 (95% CI 0.17, 1.42) • No effect on carpometacarpal joint (OR 0.94, 95% CI 0.44, 2.03)

Abbreviations: CI, confidence interval; DIP, distal interphalangeal joint; OR, odds ratio.

who had had hysterectomies (n = 10,272) were randomly assigned to receive 0.625 mg per day of conjugated equine estrogen or placebo. Those with an intact uterus (n = 16,049) were randomly assigned to receive estrogen (conjugated equine estrogen 0.625 mg) and progestin (medroxyprogesterone acetate 2.5 mg/d) versus placebo. Women receiving estrogen alone had significantly lower rates of arthroplasty (hazard ratio [HR] 0.84, 95% confidence interval [CI]: 0.70–1.00). This effect had only borderline significance for hip arthroplasty (HR 0.73, 95% CI: 0.52–1.03) and was not significant for knee arthroplasty. In the estrogen and progestin trial, there was no association for total, hip, or knee arthroplasty.[108] In a recent prospective study of 2621 women greater estradiol concentration was associated with lower incidence of knee replacement (HR 0.70, 95% CI: 0.50–0.96). Lower androstenedione concentration and higher sex hormone–binding protein concentration were associated with higher incidence of knee replacement (HR 1.7, 95% CI 1.05–2.77).[109] Estrogen seems to have a protective effect on joint replacement, specifically on the hip more than the knee; however, this effect is negated by the presence of progestin. Further studies are needed to clarify the role of estrogen after menopause on mitigating OA.

Sjögren Syndrome

Primary Sjögren syndrome has a marked bias toward women with at least a 10:1 ratio to men but generally has its onset late in life, frequently in postmenopausal years.[110] Nonetheless, menopause and its effects on this disease are little studied. Postmenopausal as well as premenopausal women with Sjögren syndrome have increased vaginal dryness and dyspareunia[111] as well as decreased quality of sexual life compared with controls.[112] The decrease was related to multiple factors, including dyspareunia, lubrication, desire, and arousal according to the Female Sexual Function Index.[112]

Sex hormone levels have been studied minimally compared with other rheumatic illnesses. One small study of 17 patients with Sjögren syndrome and 19 healthy controls showed statistically significantly higher prolactin levels among the patients (11.4 vs 6.7 ng/mL), whereas there were no statistical differences of estrogen or progesterone levels.[113] There is an aspect of sex hormone metabolism that could be affected uniquely by Sjögren syndrome among the rheumatic illnesses. Dehydroepiandrosterone-sulfate (DHEAS) is produced in the adrenal glands of estrogen-deficient women and is converted into dehydroepiandrosterone in exocrine glands. This latter metabolism may be abnormal as a result of Sjögren related dysfunction of these glands resulting in immune effects.[114,115] Trials of dehydroepiandrosterone in Sjögren syndrome have failed to show a benefit for fatigue or salivary flow even among patients with low serum levels.[116–118] Perhaps these negative trials were the result of failure to convert DHEAS in exocrine gland tissue.

Scleroderma

Systemic sclerosis (SSc) is a disorder characterized by vascular damage and overproduction of collagen and its deposition and other matrix constituents into skin and internal organs.[119] Estrogens have a protective role on arterial endothelium.[119] Postmenopausal patients with SSc have lower levels of testosterone, DHEAS, and androstenedione compared with controls. There is a negative correlation between androstenedione and anticentromere antibody (ACA) levels. It was postulated that ACA is generally present in localized SSc and a higher level of hormones suppresses the autoimmune process in the skin and synthesis of ACA. Surprisingly, the same study has shown a positive correlation between anti-topoisomerase I antibodies and androgen levels.[120]

Menopause has effects on skin thickening, especially in SSc patients with diffuse skin disease. Postmenopausal women with diffuse SSc have lower mean modified Rodnan skin scores compared with premenopausal status women. The effect was smaller, but statistically significant, in patients with limited skin disease.[121]

In contrast to the skin, postmenopausal status is a risk factor for developing pulmonary hypertension. In the study by Scorza and colleagues,[119] 93 patients (49.2%) were postmenopausal and 49 (31.2%) were fertile. The cumulative probability of pulmonary hypertension increased over time in postmenopausal women compared with fertile women. The mean free interval time for pulmonary hypertension was 10.6 years in postmenopausal subjects compared with 20 years in fertile subjects ($P<.003$). Relative risk of menopause for pulmonary hypertension was 5.2, with a P value of less than .0001. The mechanism underlying this effect was postulated as a lack of estrogen leading to a decrease in nitrous oxide production and endothelial damage. One retrospective study found that HRT soon after menopause is beneficial in preventing pulmonary hypertension in patients with limited SSc. However, the study was retrospective and the duration of hormone therapy was not defined. Randomized controlled trials are required to draw definitive conclusions.[122]

Postmenopausal women with SSc have a higher prevalence of osteoporosis (42.7%) compared with controls (10.7%), with significant alteration in the trabecular bone component in patients with SSc. The presence of ACA was associated with lower bone mineral density in the same study. Digital ulceration was associated with lower total hip and femoral neck bone density.[123] Another study pointed out that earlier onset of menopause in patients with SSc is associated with lower bone mineral density.[124]

SUMMARY

Menopause interacts with rheumatic disease in various ways. For example, SLE with onset after menopause is generally milder, whereas menopause is a risk factor for pulmonary hypertension in SSc. The data concerning the relationship of menopause and rheumatic diseases are incomplete or contradictory in many cases. Osteoporosis is a part of many of these diseases, and the risk for this complication is increased by menopause. In SLE, treatment with cyclophosphamide can cause premature menopause, especially in women older than 30 years who have decreased ovarian reserve. Treatment of menopause with hormone therapy has differential effects depending on the disease and the manifestation examined.

REFERENCES

1. Hall JE. Endocrinology of the menopause. Endocrinol Metab Clin North Am 2015;44(3):485–96.
2. Daan NM, Fauser BC. Menopause prediction and potential implications. Maturitas 2015;82(3):257–65.
3. Perls TT, Fretts RC. The evolution of menopause and human life span. Ann Hum Biol 2001;28(3):237–45.
4. Perls TT, Alpert L, Fretts RC. Middle-aged mothers live longer. Nature 1997; 389(6647):133.
5. Sievert LL. Anthropology and the study of menopause: evolutionary, developmental, and comparative perspectives. Menopause 2014;21(10):1151–9.
6. Peccei JS. A hypothesis for the origin and evolution of menopause. Maturitas 1995;21(2):83–9.

7. Peccei JS. A critique of the grandmother hypotheses: old and new. Am J Hum Biol 2001;13(4):434–52.
8. Kuhle BX. An evolutionary perspective on the origin and ontogeny of menopause. Maturitas 2007;57(4):329–37.
9. Lahdenpera M, Lummaa V, Russell AF. Menopause: why does fertility end before life? Climacteric 2004;7(4):327–31 [discussion: 331–2].
10. Lahdenpera M, Russell AF, Tremblay M, et al. Selection on menopause in two premodern human populations: no evidence for the mother hypothesis. Evolution 2011;65(2):476–89.
11. Lahdenpera M, Gillespie DO, Lummaa V, et al. Severe intergenerational reproductive conflict and the evolution of menopause. Ecol Lett 2012;15(11): 1283–90.
12. Penn DJ, Smith KR. Differential fitness costs of reproduction between the sexes. Proc Natl Acad Sci U S A 2007;104(2):553–8.
13. Shanley DP, Sear R, Mace R, et al. Testing evolutionary theories of menopause. Proc Biol Sci 2007;274(1628):2943–9.
14. Brent LJ, Franks DW, Foster EA, et al. Ecological knowledge, leadership, and the evolution of menopause in killer whales. Curr Biol 2015;25(6):746–50.
15. Johnstone RA, Cant MA. The evolution of menopause in cetaceans and humans: the role of demography. Proc Biol Sci 2010;277(1701):3765–71.
16. Borchers AT, Naguwa SM, Shoenfeld Y, et al. The geoepidemiology of systemic lupus erythematosus. Autoimmun Rev 2010;9(5):A277–87.
17. Alpizar-Rodriguez D, Romero-Diaz J, Sanchez-Guerrero J, et al. Age at natural menopause among patients with systemic lupus erythematosus. Rheumatology (Oxford) 2014;53(11):2023–9.
18. Gonzalez LA, Pons-Estel GJ, Zhang JS, et al. Effect of age, menopause and cyclophosphamide use on damage accrual in systemic lupus erythematosus patients from LUMINA, a multiethnic US cohort (LUMINA LXIII). Lupus 2009; 18(2):184–6.
19. Ioannidis JP, Katsifis GE, Tzioufas AG, et al. Predictors of sustained amenorrhea from pulsed intravenous cyclophosphamide in premenopausal women with systemic lupus erythematosus. J Rheumatol 2002;29(10):2129–35.
20. Laskari K, Zintzaras E, Tzioufas AG. Ovarian function is preserved in women with severe systemic lupus erythematosus after a 6-month course of cyclophosphamide followed by mycophenolate mofetil. Clin Exp Rheumatol 2010;28(1):83–6.
21. McDermott EM, Powell RJ. Incidence of ovarian failure in systemic lupus erythematosus after treatment with pulse cyclophosphamide. Ann Rheum Dis 1996; 55(4):224–9.
22. Medeiros MM, Silveira VA, Menezes AP, et al. Risk factors for ovarian failure in patients with systemic lupus erythematosus. Braz J Med Biol Res 2001; 34(12):1561–8.
23. Lawrenz B, Henes J, Henes M, et al. Impact of systemic lupus erythematosus on ovarian reserve in premenopausal women: evaluation by using anti-Muellerian hormone. Lupus 2011;20(11):1193–7.
24. Morel N, Bachelot A, Chakhtoura Z, et al. Study of anti-mullerian hormone and its relation to the subsequent probability of pregnancy in 112 patients with systemic lupus erythematosus, exposed or not to cyclophosphamide. J Clin Endocrinol Metab 2013;98(9):3785–92.
25. Pasoto SG, Viana VS, Mendonca BB, et al. Anti-corpus luteum antibody: a novel serological marker for ovarian dysfunction in systemic lupus erythematosus? J Rheumatol 1999;26(5):1087–93.

26. Mayorga J, Alpizar-Rodriguez D, Prieto-Padilla J, et al. Prevalence of premature ovarian failure in patients with systemic lupus erythematosus. Lupus 2016;25(7): 675–83.
27. Marder W, McCune WJ, Wang L, et al. Adjunctive GnRH-a treatment attenuates depletion of ovarian reserve associated with cyclophosphamide therapy in premenopausal SLE patients. Gynecol Endocrinol 2012;28(8):624–7.
28. Brunner HI, Silva CA, Reiff A, et al. Randomized, double-blind, dose-escalation trial of triptorelin for ovary protection in childhood-onset systemic lupus erythematosus. Arthritis Rheumatol 2015;67(5):1377–85.
29. Oktem O, Guzel Y, Aksoy S, et al. Ovarian function and reproductive outcomes of female patients with systemic lupus erythematosus and the strategies to preserve their fertility. Obstet Gynecol Surv 2015;70(3):196–210.
30. Deng XL, Liu XY. Less disease severity and favorable prognosis are associated with postmenopausal systemic lupus erythematosus patients. Rheumatol Int 2009;29(5):535–8.
31. Lazaro D. Elderly-onset systemic lupus erythematosus: prevalence, clinical course and treatment. Drugs Aging 2007;24(9):701–15.
32. Mok CC, Lau CS, Ho CT, et al. Do flares of systemic lupus erythematosus decline after menopause? Scand J Rheumatol 1999;28(6):357–62.
33. Sanchez-Guerrero J, Villegas A, Mendoza-Fuentes A, et al. Disease activity during the premenopausal and postmenopausal periods in women with systemic lupus erythematosus. Am J Med 2001;111(6):464–8.
34. Namjou B, Scofield RH, Kelly JA, et al. The effects of previous hysterectomy on lupus. Lupus 2009;18(11):1000–5.
35. Urowitz MB, Ibanez D, Jerome D, et al. The effect of menopause on disease activity in systemic lupus erythematosus. J Rheumatol 2006;33(11):2192–8.
36. Rojas-Villarraga A, Torres-Gonzalez JV, Ruiz-Sternberg AM. Safety of hormonal replacement therapy and oral contraceptives in systemic lupus erythematosus: a systematic review and meta-analysis. PLoS One 2014;9(8):e104303.
37. Khafagy AM, Stewart KI, Christianson MS, et al. Effect of menopause hormone therapy on disease progression in systemic lupus erythematosus: a systematic review. Maturitas 2015;81(2):276–81.
38. Sanchez-Guerrero J, Liang MH, Karlson EW, et al. Postmenopausal estrogen therapy and the risk for developing systemic lupus erythematosus. Ann Intern Med 1995;122(6):430–3.
39. Buyon JP, Petri MA, Kim MY, et al. The effect of combined estrogen and progesterone hormone replacement therapy on disease activity in systemic lupus erythematosus: a randomized trial. Ann Intern Med 2005;142(12 Pt 1):953–62.
40. Klonowska-Szymczyk A, Wolska A, Robak T, et al. Expression of toll-like receptors 3, 7, and 9 in peripheral blood mononuclear cells from patients with systemic lupus erythematosus. Mediators Inflamm 2014;2014:381418.
41. Evans MJ, MacLaughlin S, Marvin RD, et al. Estrogen decreases in vitro apoptosis of peripheral blood mononuclear cells from women with normal menstrual cycles and decreases TNF-alpha production in SLE but not in normal cultures. Clin Immunol Immunopathol 1997;82(3):258–62.
42. Lee C, Almagor O, Dunlop DD, et al. Disease damage and low bone mineral density: an analysis of women with systemic lupus erythematosus ever and never receiving corticosteroids. Rheumatology (Oxford) 2006;45(1):53–60.
43. Mendoza-Pinto C, Garcia-Carrasco M, Sandoval-Cruz H, et al. Risk factors of vertebral fractures in women with systemic lupus erythematosus. Clin Rheumatol 2009;28(5):579–85.

44. Mak A, Lim JQ, Liu Y, et al. Significantly higher estimated 10-year probability of fracture in lupus patients with bone mineral density comparable to that of healthy individuals. Rheumatol Int 2013;33(2):299–307.

45. Mok CC, To CH, Mak A, et al. Raloxifene for postmenopausal women with systemic lupus erythematosus: a pilot randomized controlled study. Arthritis Rheum 2005;52(12):3997–4002.

46. Mok CC, Ying SK, Ma KM, et al. Effect of raloxifene on disease activity and vascular biomarkers in patients with systemic lupus erythematosus: subgroup analysis of a double-blind randomized controlled trial. Lupus 2013;22(14): 1470–8.

47. Ward MM, Pyun E, Studenski S. Long-term survival in systemic lupus erythematosus. Patient characteristics associated with poorer outcomes. Arthritis Rheum 1995;38(2):274–83.

48. Ribeiro GG, Bonfa E, Sasdeli Neto R, et al. Premature coronary artery calcification is associated with disease duration and bone mineral density in young female systemic lupus erythematosus patients. Lupus 2010;19(1):27–33.

49. Selzer F, Sutton-Tyrrell K, Fitzgerald S, et al. Vascular stiffness in women with systemic lupus erythematosus. Hypertension 2001;37(4):1075–82.

50. Mak A, Liu Y, Ho RC. Endothelium-dependent but not endothelium-independent flow-mediated dilation is significantly reduced in patients with systemic lupus erythematosus without vascular events: a metaanalysis and metaregression. J Rheumatol 2011;38(7):1296–303.

51. Santos MJ, Pedro LM, Canhao H, et al. Hemorheological parameters are related to subclinical atherosclerosis in systemic lupus erythematosus and rheumatoid arthritis patients. Atherosclerosis 2011;219(2):821–6.

52. Barragan-Martinez C, Amaya-Amaya J, Pineda-Tamayo R, et al. Gender differences in Latin-American patients with rheumatoid arthritis. Gend Med 2012; 9(6):490–510.e5.

53. Goemaere S, Ackerman C, Goethals K, et al. Onset of symptoms of rheumatoid arthritis in relation to age, sex and menopausal transition. J Rheumatol 1990; 17(12):1620–2.

54. Gabriel SE. The epidemiology of rheumatoid arthritis. Rheum Dis Clin North Am 2001;27(2):269–81.

55. Carette S, Marcoux S, Gingras S. Postmenopausal hormones and the incidence of rheumatoid arthritis. J Rheumatol 1989;16(7):911–3.

56. Linos A, Worthington JW, O'Fallon WM, et al. Case-control study of rheumatoid arthritis and prior use of oral contraceptives. Lancet 1983;1(8337):1299–300.

57. Pikwer M, Nilsson JA, Bergstrom U, et al. Early menopause and severity of rheumatoid arthritis in women older than 45 years. Arthritis Res Ther 2012;14(4): R190.

58. Beydoun HA, el-Amin R, McNeal M, et al. Reproductive history and postmenopausal rheumatoid arthritis among women 60 years or older: third national health and nutrition examination survey. Menopause 2013;20(9):930–5.

59. Criswell LA, Merlino LA, Cerhan JR, et al. Cigarette smoking and the risk of rheumatoid arthritis among postmenopausal women: results from the Iowa Women's Health Study. Am J Med 2002;112(6):465–71.

60. Krishnan E, Sokka T, Hannonen P. Smoking-gender interaction and risk for rheumatoid arthritis. Arthritis Res Ther 2003;5(3):R158–62.

61. Hernandez-Avila M, Liang MH, Willett WC, et al. Oral contraceptives, replacement oestrogens and the risk of rheumatoid arthritis. Br J Rheumatol 1989; 28(Suppl 1):31 [discussion: 42–5].

62. Hazes JM, Dijkmans BC, Vandenbroucke JP, et al. Reduction of the risk of rheumatoid arthritis among women who take oral contraceptives. Arthritis Rheum 1990;33(2):173–9.
63. Linos A, Kaklamanis E, Kontomerkos A, et al. Rheumatoid arthritis and oral contraceptives in the Greek female population: a case-control study. Br J Rheumatol 1989;28(Suppl 1):37 [discussion: 42–5].
64. Vandenbroucke JP, Witteman JC, Valkenburg HA, et al. Noncontraceptive hormones and rheumatoid arthritis in perimenopausal and postmenopausal women. JAMA 1986;255(10):1299–303.
65. Koepsell TD, Dugowson CE, Nelson JL, et al. Non-contraceptive hormones and the risk of rheumatoid arthritis in menopausal women. Int J Epidemiol 1994; 23(6):1248–55.
66. Orellana C, Saevarsdottir S, Klareskog L, et al. Postmenopausal hormone therapy and the risk of rheumatoid arthritis: results from the Swedish EIRA population-based case-control study. Eur J Epidemiol 2015;30(5):449–57.
67. Wluka AE, Cicuttini FM, Spector TD. Menopause, oestrogens and arthritis. Maturitas 2000;35(3):183–99.
68. Salliot C, Bombardier C, Saraux A, et al. Hormonal replacement therapy may reduce the risk for RA in women with early arthritis who carry HLA-DRB1 01 and/or 04 alleles by protecting against the production of anti-CCP: results from the ESPOIR cohort. Ann Rheum Dis 2010;69(9):1683–6.
69. Islander U, Jochems C, Lagerquist MK, et al. Estrogens in rheumatoid arthritis; the immune system and bone. Mol Cell Endocrinol 2011;335(1):14–29.
70. d'Elia HF, Carlsten H. The impact of hormone replacement therapy on humoral and cell-mediated immune responses in vivo in post-menopausal women with rheumatoid arthritis. Scand J Immunol 2008;68(6):661–7.
71. Hall GM, Daniels M, Huskisson EC, et al. A randomised controlled trial of the effect of hormone replacement therapy on disease activity in postmenopausal rheumatoid arthritis. Ann Rheum Dis 1994;53(2):112–6.
72. Aeberli D, Schett G. Cortical remodeling during menopause, rheumatoid arthritis, glucocorticoid and bisphosphonate therapy. Arthritis Res Ther 2013; 15(2):208.
73. Oelzner P, Schwabe A, Lehmann G, et al. Significance of risk factors for osteoporosis is dependent on gender and menopause in rheumatoid arthritis. Rheumatol Int 2008;28(11):1143–50.
74. Lee SG, Park YE, Park SH, et al. Increased frequency of osteoporosis and BMD below the expected range for age among South Korean women with rheumatoid arthritis. Int J Rheum Dis 2012;15(3):289–96.
75. Kroot EJ, Nieuwenhuizen MG, de Waal Malefijt MC, et al. Change in bone mineral density in patients with rheumatoid arthritis during the first decade of the disease. Arthritis Rheum 2001;44(6):1254–60.
76. Hauser B, Riches PL, Wilson JF, et al. Prevalence and clinical prediction of osteoporosis in a contemporary cohort of patients with rheumatoid arthritis. Rheumatology (Oxford) 2014;53(10):1759–66.
77. Hall GM, Spector TD, Delmas PD. Markers of bone metabolism in postmenopausal women with rheumatoid arthritis. Effects of corticosteroids and hormone replacement therapy. Arthritis Rheum 1995;38(7):902–6.
78. Als OS, Riis BJ, Gotfredsen A, et al. Biochemical markers of bone turnover in rheumatoid arthritis. Relation to anti-inflammatory treatment, sex, and menopause. Acta Med Scand 1986;219(2):209–13.

79. Myasoedova E, Davis JM 3rd, Crowson CS, et al. Epidemiology of rheumatoid arthritis: rheumatoid arthritis and mortality. Curr Rheumatol Rep 2010;12(5): 379–85.
80. Meek IL, Vonkeman HE, van de Laar MA. Cardiovascular case fatality in rheumatoid arthritis is decreasing; first prospective analysis of a current low disease activity rheumatoid arthritis cohort and review of the literature. BMC Musculoskelet Disord 2014;15:142.
81. Kuller LH, Mackey RH, Walitt BT, et al. Determinants of mortality among postmenopausal women in the women's health initiative who report rheumatoid arthritis. Arthritis Rheumatol 2014;66(3):497–507 [Erratum appears in Arthritis Rheumatol 2014;66(5):1394].
82. Solomon DH, Curhan GC, Rimm EB, et al. Cardiovascular risk factors in women with and without rheumatoid arthritis. Arthritis Rheum 2004;50(11):3444–9.
83. Mackey RH, Kuller LH, Deane KD, et al. Rheumatoid arthritis, anti-cyclic citrullinated peptide positivity, and cardiovascular disease risk in the women's health initiative. Arthritis Rheumatol 2015;67(9):2311–22.
84. Park YB, Ahn CW, Choi HK, et al. Atherosclerosis in rheumatoid arthritis: morphologic evidence obtained by carotid ultrasound. Arthritis Rheum 2002; 46(7):1714–9.
85. Inaba M, Tanaka K, Goto H, et al. Independent association of increased trunk fat with increased arterial stiffening in postmenopausal patients with rheumatoid arthritis. J Rheumatol 2007;34(2):290–5.
86. Wright NC, Riggs GK, Lisse JR, et al. Self-reported osteoarthritis, ethnicity, body mass index, and other associated risk factors in postmenopausal women-results from the women's health initiative. J Am Geriatr Soc 2008;56(9):1736–43.
87. Multanen J, Heinonen A, Hakkinen A, et al. Bone and cartilage characteristics in postmenopausal women with mild knee radiographic osteoarthritis and those without radiographic osteoarthritis. J Musculoskelet Neuronal Interact 2015; 15(1):69–77.
88. Arden NK, Griffiths GO, Hart DJ, et al. The association between osteoarthritis and osteoporotic fracture: the Chingford Study. Br J Rheumatol 1996;35(12): 1299–304.
89. Arden NK, Crozier S, Smith H, et al. Knee pain, knee osteoarthritis, and the risk of fracture. Arthritis Rheum 2006;55(4):610–5.
90. Smith TO, Higson E, Pearson M, et al. Is there an increased risk of falls and fractures in people with early diagnosed hip and knee osteoarthritis? Data from the osteoarthritis initiative. Int J Rheum Dis 2016. [Epub ahead of print].
91. Vestergaard P, Rejnmark L, Mosekilde L. Osteoarthritis and risk of fractures. Calcif Tissue Int 2009;84(4):249–56.
92. Martin-Millan M, Castaneda S. Estrogens, osteoarthritis and inflammation. Joint Bone Spine 2013;80(4):368–73.
93. Tinti L, Niccolini S, Lamboglia A, et al. Raloxifene protects cultured human chondrocytes from IL-1beta induced damage: a biochemical and morphological study. Eur J Pharmacol 2011;670(1):67–73.
94. Riancho JA, Garcia-Ibarbia C, Gravani A, et al. Common variations in estrogen-related genes are associated with severe large-joint osteoarthritis: a multicenter genetic and functional study. Osteoarthritis Cartilage 2010;18(7):927–33.
95. Ma H, Wu W, Yang X, et al. Genetic effects of common polymorphisms in estrogen receptor alpha gene on osteoarthritis: a meta-analysis. Int J Clin Exp Med 2015;8(8):13446–54.

96. Bay-Jensen AC, Tabassi NC, Sondergaard LV, et al. The response to oestrogen deprivation of the cartilage collagen degradation marker, CTX-II, is unique compared with other markers of collagen turnover. Arthritis Res Ther 2009;11(1):R9.
97. Lou C, Xiang G, Weng Q, et al. Menopause is associated with articular cartilage degeneration: a clinical study of knee joint in 860 women. Menopause 2016; 23(11):1239–46.
98. Tsai CL, Liu TK. Estradiol-induced knee osteoarthrosis in ovariectomized rabbits. Clin Orthop Relat Res 1993;291:295–302.
99. Richette P, Dumontier MF, Francois M, et al. Dual effects of 17beta-oestradiol on interleukin 1beta-induced proteoglycan degradation in chondrocytes. Ann Rheum Dis 2004;63(2):191–9.
100. Gao W, Zeng C, Cai D, et al. Serum concentrations of selected endogenous estrogen and estrogen metabolites in pre- and post-menopausal Chinese women with osteoarthritis. J Endocrinol Invest 2010;33(9):644–9.
101. Gao WL, Wu LS, Zi JH, et al. Measurement of serum estrogen and estrogen metabolites in pre- and postmenopausal women with osteoarthritis using high-performance liquid chromatography-electrospray ionization-tandem mass spectrometry. Braz J Med Biol Res 2015;48(2):146–53.
102. Parazzini F, Progretto Menopausa Italia Study Group. Menopausal status, hormone replacement therapy use and risk of self-reported physician-diagnosed osteoarthritis in women attending menopause clinics in Italy. Maturitas 2003; 46(3):207–12.
103. Von Mühlen D, Morton D, Von Muhlen CA, et al. Postmenopausal estrogen and increased risk of clinical osteoarthritis at the hip, hand, and knee in older women. J Womens Health Gend Based Med 2002;11(6):511–8.
104. Nevitt MC, Cummings SR, Lane NE, et al. Association of estrogen replacement therapy with the risk of osteoarthritis of the hip in elderly white women. Study of Osteoporotic Fractures Research Group. Arch Intern Med 1996;156(18): 2073–80.
105. Hannan MT, Felson DT, Anderson JJ, et al. Estrogen use and radiographic osteoarthritis of the knee in women. The Framingham Osteoarthritis Study. Arthritis Rheum Apr 1990;33(4):525–32.
106. Nevitt MC, Felson DT, Williams EN, et al. The effect of estrogen plus progestin on knee symptoms and related disability in postmenopausal women: the Heart and Estrogen/Progestin Replacement Study, a randomized, double-blind, placebo-controlled trial. Arthritis Rheum Apr 2001;44(4):811–8.
107. Spector TD, Nandra D, Hart DJ, et al. Is hormone replacement therapy protective for hand and knee osteoarthritis in women?: The Chingford Study. Ann Rheum Dis 1997;56(7):432–4.
108. Cirillo DJ, Wallace RB, Wu L, et al. Effect of hormone therapy on risk of hip and knee joint replacement in the women's health initiative. Arthritis Rheum 2006; 54(10):3194–204.
109. Hussain SM, Cicuttini FM, Bell RJ, et al. Incidence of total knee and hip replacement for osteoarthritis in relation to circulating sex steroid hormone concentrations in women. Arthritis Rheumatol 2014;66(8):2144–51.
110. Qin B, Wang J, Yang Z, et al. Epidemiology of primary Sjögren's syndrome: a systematic review and meta-analysis. Ann Rheum Dis 2015;74(11):1983–9.
111. Marchesoni D, Mozzanega B, De Sandre P, et al. Gynaecological aspects of primary Sjögren's syndrome. Eur J Obstet Gynecol Reprod Biol 1995;63(1):49–53.
112. Priori R, Minniti A, Derme M, et al. Quality of sexual life in women with primary Sjögren syndrome. J Rheumatol 2015;42(8):1427–31.

113. Taiym S, Haghighat N, Al-Hashimi I. A comparison of the hormone levels in patients with Sjögren's syndrome and healthy controls. Oral Surg Oral Med Oral Pathol Oral Radiol Endod 2004;97(5):579–83.

114. Konttinen YT, Fuellen G, Bing Y, et al. Sex steroids in Sjögren's syndrome. J Autoimmun 2012;39(1–2):49–56.

115. Konttinen YT, Stegajev V, Al-Samadi A, et al. Sjögren's syndrome and extragonadal sex steroid formation: a clue to a better disease control? J Steroid Biochem Mol Biol 2015;145:237–44.

116. Porola P, Straub RH, Virkki LM, et al. Failure of oral DHEA treatment to increase local salivary androgen outputs of female patients with Sjögren's syndrome. Scand J Rheumatol 2011;40(5):387–90.

117. Virkki LM, Porola P, Forsblad-d'Elia H, et al. Dehydroepiandrosterone (DHEA) substitution treatment for severe fatigue in DHEA-deficient patients with primary Sjögren's syndrome. Arthritis Care Res 2010;62(1):118–24.

118. Hartkamp A, Geenen R, Godaert GL, et al. Effect of dehydroepiandrosterone administration on fatigue, well-being, and functioning in women with primary Sjögren syndrome: a randomised controlled trial. Ann Rheum Dis 2008;67(1):91–7.

119. Scorza R, Caronni M, Bazzi S, et al. Post-menopause is the main risk factor for developing isolated pulmonary hypertension in systemic sclerosis. Ann N Y Acad Sci 2002;966:238–46.

120. Perkovic D, Martinovic Kaliterna D, Jurisic Z, et al. Androgens in postmenopausal patients with systemic sclerosis. Rheumatology (Oxford) 2015; 54(4):744–6.

121. Vinet E, Bernatsky S, Hudson M, et al. Effect of menopause on the modified Rodnan skin score in systemic sclerosis. Arthritis Res Ther 2014;16(3):R130.

122. Beretta L, Caronni M, Origgi L, et al. Hormone replacement therapy may prevent the development of isolated pulmonary hypertension in patients with systemic sclerosis and limited cutaneous involvement. Scand J Rheumatol 2006;35:468–71.

123. Marot M, Valery A, Esteve E, et al. Prevalence and predictive factors of osteoporosis in systemic sclerosis patients: a case-control study. Oncotarget 2015; 6(17):14865–73.

124. La Montagna G, Vatti M, Valentini G, et al. Osteopenia in systemic sclerosis. Evidence of a participating role of earlier menopause. Clin Rheumatol 1991;10(1): 18–22.

Index

Note: Page numbers of article titles are in **boldface** type.

Rheum Dis Clin N Am 43 (2017) 303–312
http://dx.doi.org/10.1016/S0889-857X(17)30010-8
0889-857X/17

rheumatic.theclinics.com

Moving?

Make sure your subscription moves with you!

To notify us of your new address, find your **Clinics Account Number** (located on your mailing label above your name), and contact customer service at:

Email: journalscustomerservice-usa@elsevier.com

800-654-2452 (subscribers in the U.S. & Canada)
314-447-8871 (subscribers outside of the U.S. & Canada)

Fax number: 314-447-8029

Elsevier Health Sciences Division
Subscription Customer Service
3251 Riverport Lane
Maryland Heights, MO 63043

*To ensure uninterrupted delivery of your subscription, please notify us at least 4 weeks in advance of move.

Printed and bound by CPI Group (UK) Ltd, Croydon, CR0 4YY

08/05/2025

01864699-0007